Scissors Skills

Scissors Skills

DOROTHY E PENSO Dip COT, FAETC

Paediatric Occupational Therapist

W

WHURR PUBLISHERS

LONDON

© 2004 Whurr Publishers
Whurr Publishers Ltd
19b Compton Terrace, London N1 2UN, England

British Library Cataloguing in Publication Data
A catalogue record for this book is available from the British Library.

ISBN 1 86156 423 6

Printed and bound in the UK by Athenaeum Press Ltd, Gateshead, Tyne & Wear

Contents

Acknowledgements

Throughout my career as a paediatric occupational therapist I have helped many children and adults to develop scissors skills. They have taught me to understand their difficulties when using scissors and how best to develop strategies to help them. I thank all those people who have provided me with the basis for this book.

A number of illustrations have appeared in two of my previous books, Occupational Therapy for Children with Disabilities (1987) and Perceptuo-motor Difficulties, Theory and Strategies to Help Children, Adolescents and Adults (1993) and appear with permission of Nelson Thornes Ltd.

Illustrations of some special types of scissors have been kindly provided by Peta (UK) Ltd, Mark's Hall, Mark's Hall Lane, Margaret Roding, Dunmow, CM6 1QT. Luisa Dilella of the Early Learning Centre provided the illustration of children's left-handed scissors. Joanna and Alice Penso helped by posing for the illustrations of sitting positions and cutting with scissors.

CHAPTER 1

Introduction

Scissors have been known for many centuries. One of the earliest surviving pairs was found in Egypt and dates back to 300BC. At about the same time, Italian shepherds used scissors to shear sheep (Armada Art 1998). These so-called scissors were probably more like shears which required both hands to use them. The first cross-bladed scissors were used in Rome in 100AD. The first written evidence of scissors was made by the scribe Isadore of Seville in 500AD. It was not until the 16th century that scissors came into domestic use in Europe.

The term 'scissors' originated in late medieval English, equated with old French 'cisoires', which is now only used to describe large shears. Both terms originate from Latin 'cisorium', cutting instrument. The Shorter Oxford English Dictionary describes scissors thus:

> *A cutting instrument consisting of a pair of handled blades, so pivoted on a pin in the centre that the instrument can be opened to a shape resembling that of the letter X, and the handles then brought together again so as to cause the edges of the blades to close on the object to be cut.*

This description of the functioning of scissors illustrates the hand movement required to operate them, that is, the apposition of the thumb to the fingers. Unlike shears, scissors are operated by one hand. (Some small children have been seen to try to use scissors as shears, holding one of the handles in each hand.)

It is difficult to imagine life without scissors. Until their invention, clothes must have consisted of draped lengths of material for it would have been extremely difficult to cut woven fabric into more complex shapes. Before scissors were available the only way to cut hair would be with a blade. How were finger- and toenails trimmed? (The author has seen old men 'paring' their nails with a penknife!) How were intricate shapes cut out of paper and other materials? Scissors are important in professions such as bespoke tailoring, dressmaking, upholstery, wallpaper hanging and hairdressing, and to a lesser extent in many other professions.

Today almost every home has at least one pair of scissors, which most people would consider to be indispensable for cutting paper, card and fabrics. In the kitchen some people use scissors rather than a knife for cutting, slicing and chopping some foods. Today scissors are manufactured for numerous specific uses from cutting embroidery thread to cutting cardboard. Special scissors are manufactured for cutting and thinning hair. Scissors which produce a fancy cut edge are manufactured for use in various paper crafts and pinking shears are used to finish the edges of non-fray fabrics.

It is only in comparatively recent years that attention has been given to the complexities of using scissors effectively. Cutting with scissors can be one of the most complex hand skills we undertake. It is a two-handed activity in which each hand must move accurately and independently, each performing a quite different type of movement; one hand manipulating the scissors while the other hand manoeuvres the material being cut. In addition there must be constant visual monitoring of the task, not of the motion of the scissors or the hand holding the material being cut. Using scissors requires concentration, and sometimes meticulous care, where precise cutting is required.

Scissors hold a fascination for most young children. Initially they will attempt to cut almost any material with them, sometimes their own hair! Most young children take joy in snipping paper and later, as the skill develops, many enjoy cutting out shapes and figures. During early school years cutting with scissors forms a large part of art and craft activities, especially before festivals such as Christmas, Easter and other celebrations. As children progress to secondary school there is less opportunity to use scissors skills except for periods of craftwork.

Throughout life there are times when scissors skills are needed and where their inefficient use will lead to frustration and irritation and sometimes self-damage. Scissors skills may never have been mastered due to lack of opportunity or poor teaching. For some people difficulties in using scissors may be the result of a life-long disability and for others the result of disease or disability acquired later in life. Such problems may be developmental, sensory, motor or perceptual, or may be caused by lack of muscle power, neurological abnormalities, mechanical limitations or be due to pain or swelling of the hands or fingers.

With help in the appropriate choice of scissors from the wide range which is available today, and guidance in their use, most children and adults can achieve skills which bring a degree of pleasure, satisfaction and success.

This book provides strategies and suggestions to help both children and adults. There are discussion and suggestions of the skills needed to use scissors effectively. There is reference to some conditions which may delay or preclude the acquisition of these skills. Special scissors may be required for people with certain conditions, in order for those people to cut effectively. As with all fine motor activities it is important to consider trunk stability and overall position both with regards to safety and efficiency. Descriptions and illustrations are provided of the features of the various types of scissors which are available. A further chapter considers pre-scissors activities intended to promote all aspects of scissors skills. There is a section of scissors activities which are carefully graded so that choices may be made to suit most levels and speeds of learning. These graded activities are supported by an appendix of photocopiable worksheets of various levels of activities.

The book will be a much used addition to the book shelves of occupational therapy and rehabilitation departments and individual therapists. Teachers at all stages of education will find it useful, as will classroom support assistants. It follows that it should be available in the libraries of colleges and universities which have faculties of occupational therapy and education. In fact anyone who needs to use scissors, or teach others to use them, will find that the book contains pertinent information.

CHAPTER 2

Skills needed to use scissors effectively

Many skills are combined in order to cut with scissors. The first of these skills is perhaps the desire and motivation to use scissors to produce some effect or change in the material being cut. This presumes a degree of pre-knowledge of the uses and possibilities of what may be achieved with scissors. If there is no pre-knowledge of scissors, demonstrations and discussion will be necessary to promote motivation and stimulate desire to learn scissors skills.

Learning and using any motor skill involves the use of much more than movement. A whole chain of events must take place before there is motor effect (Figure 2.1).

Sensory input

The senses, particularly vision and touch, are important when undertaking scissors activities. The eyes see the material to be cut and the scissors, or other cutting tool, to be used. Judgement must be used to ensure that the scissors are in line with what is to be cut and not with the hand holding the material to be cut! Vision must be used to monitor the line on which the scissors are currently focused; any changes in the direction of the cutting must be anticipated. A sense of touch and pressure allows the user of the scissors to be aware of exactly how the scissors are being held and manipulated. In order not to damage the material being cut, the fingers must be able to sense that material and hold it with the required amount of pressure.

Perception

Information gathered from the senses is perceived; it is understood and assimilated. It is difficult to examine perception in isolation although a number of aspects of perception have been described.

Figure 2.1 Diagrammatic representation of the process from sensory input to motor output, illustrating the areas in which there may be problems.

(First appeared in: Penso DE (1993) Perceptuo-motor difficulties: theory and strategies to help children, adolescents and adults. Chapman & Hall. Reproduced by permission of Nelson Thornes Ltd.)

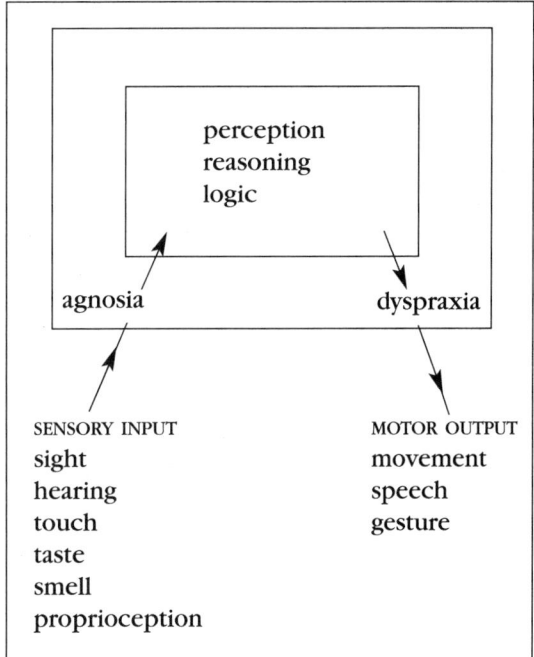

Body image

Body image describes the internal concept which we all have of our own physical configuration. This concept develops from very early infancy. Through movement, vision and proprioception, babies begin to appreciate their own body schema. They regard their hands, put them in their mouths and may have the painful experience of biting themselves. At a few months of age, a baby lying on his back sees a foot looming above and beyond his tummy, he reaches out a hand and grasps the foot and has the sensation of being held by a hand. Gradually a baby learns that he has a leg at each lower corner of himself. The young mobile child will attempt to fit herself into impossibly small spaces and will eventually learn her size: her height, width and girth. Thus body image develops.

Along with body image, there are two other closely related concepts: body schema and body awareness. Body schema develops from a child's experience of sensory information from physical movement. Body awareness is said to be dependent on the development of body schema and must be present in order for body image to develop (Williams 1983). Other perceptual skills are based on body awareness and body image.

Spatial skills

Spatial skills include appreciation of one's own position in space and the relationship of self to objects in the environment. This may be regarded in vertical, horizontal and diagonal planes, and includes the appreciation of depth. For example, when in the process of sitting on a chair, unless there is a difficulty with depth perception, it is easy to judge the depth of even an unfamiliar chair and to adopt a sitting position smoothly. The eyes are used to appreciate the height of the chair seat and often the sense of touch in the backs of the legs on the edge of the seat is an additional input which helps depth perception.

Other aspects include the appreciation of the relationship of objects to each other in both two and three dimensions, and dynamic spatial skills where there must be perception of movement. All the aspects of spatial perception play their part in scissors skills. It is, for example, important to appreciate the relationship of the blades of the scissors to the material which is being cut and to the fingers holding that material. Because the blades of the scissors are moving as well as the whole scissors progressing along the cutting line, dynamic spatial skills also play their part.

Figure/background discrimination

Figure/background discrimination can involve an aspect of perception of any of the senses; it involves extracting pertinent detail from a background containing irrelevant or distracting material. For example, in a classroom there may be sounds from outside the window, sounds of others opening bags and satchels and a murmur of other people talking, yet it is possible for most people to attend to what the teacher is saying and ignore irrelevant noises. In a visual mode there may be pictures and diagrams on the wall, books and pens on tables and a neighbouring pupil doodling with a pen, yet most people are able to attend to the diagram which the teacher is discussing. In cutting out one figure from a page of figures it is important to be able to concentrate on the relevant one. Similarly when cutting out a single complex shape, concentration must be focused on the portion of the shape which is currently being cut.

Form constancy

Form constancy is the ability to appreciate that particular objects have constant properties. A chair can take many forms; it may be for dining, rocking, reclining, having hair cut and many other uses, but all chairs have the constant property of being used for sitting on. Similarly scissors may be large or small, left-handed or right-handed, intended for cutting nails, hair, paper, fabric, food and other materials. All scissors have constant properties: there are two blades and handles usually arranged in an x configuration and they are used for cutting.

Testing perception

Various tests have been devised to test these and other aspects of perception, some of which have little or no motor aspect (Gardner 1992; Gardner 1996) and others which require a motor response (Beery and Buktenica 1997). It is possible to ascertain that information from the senses has reached the brain but far more difficult to 'observe' perception.

Motor effect

Evidence that perception has taken place is most often seen by the resultant motor effect; movement of some kind, either voluntary or involuntary. For the purposes of this study, the motor effect is the motor planning and movement necessary to use the scissors and manipulate the paper or other material effectively. Motor planning, also known as praxis, must take place before movement can be effected. Inability to plan movements mentally is known as apraxia. Difficulty with motor planning is known as dyspraxia. Following this mental unconscious planning, movement takes place. This is a gross simplification of what is an extremely complex process or sequence of events. Motor planning is essentially a neurological process and is clearly not the only process to be considered for motor function.

The ability to coordinate hand and eye is one of the major skills needed to be able to cut along lines and to cut out shapes accurately and neatly. It is important to note that the eye must be monitoring the process of cutting and *not* the movements of the scissors, which are effecting the cutting, nor the adjustments of the hand, which is holding the material which is being cut. Thus the three activities, namely those of manipulating the scissors, holding the material which is being cut and the eyes monitoring the cutting, combine to form the activity of cutting with scissors. For the eyes to be able to concentrate on the task of cutting, the process of opening and closing the blades of the scissors whilst cutting must be carried out unconsciously. The reciprocal movements of the hand to open and close the scissors must be automatic and take place without visual monitoring.

The actual manipulation of the scissors requires the ability to hold the handles or the loop of whole hand grip scissors and open and close the blades. The hand must be stabilized by the arm, which in turn is affected by the shoulder girdle and, indeed, the whole trunk. Trunk stability is also required to support the neck and the head so that the eyes may be coordinated with the hand. The shoulder girdle is attached to the trunk, and stability will enable the arm to be controlled and the hand to be sustained in an appropriate position.

Muscle power, grading of movement and mechanical difficulties caused by deformity or joint limitation also affect hand movements and consequently their quality and quantity. The degree of power and strength required will vary according to the type of cutting task. Clearly it will be easier to cut thin card rather than heavy cardboard, a light cotton fabric will be easier to cut than a heavy woollen bouclé fabric. The quality and type of the scissors being used will affect the amount of effort required. Heavy scissors such as dressmaker's shears are comparatively heavy to hold in a specific position and require considerable muscle power to open and close the blades. In contrast, small well balanced scissors intended for cutting thread are light to hold and require little power to open and close the blades. Using the type of scissors which are designed for a particular task will facilitate ease of use. Whilst not advocating the provision of dangerously sharp scissors, they must be sufficiently sharp for the task for which they are being used. Particularly in group situations such as schools it is easy to continue using scissors without checking their sharpness. Sometimes, if scissors have been misused, parts of the blade may be blunt or damaged or their alignment may be impaired. All these deficiencies will result in extra effort being needed to use the scissors, and poor results lead to frustration and reluctance to attempt similar tasks in the future.

To use conventional scissors effectively the fingers and thumb movements must be synchronized and be capable of smooth repeated reciprocal movements. These movements need to be performed without conscious motor planning and be sustained for as long as the task requires. The non-scissor hand should be able to hold the material being cut and move the material as necessary so it is cut effectively. This activity of the hand holding the material being cut should be capable of being undertaken without visual monitoring, leaving the eyes free to monitor, not the hands, but the process of cutting. Thus the activity of both hands should take place without conscious motor planning.

To use scissors effectively there must be bilateral integration. Each hand must be able to perform its individual task simultaneously and adjust its movements to suit those of the other hand. For example, the speed at which the material being cut is adjusted in the non-scissors hand will depend on the speed and positional adjustment of the scissors. Only when this skill is sufficiently mature will sophisticated cutting with scissors be able to take place.

Intellectual skills

A number of intellectual skills are also required which include the perceptual skills already described. There must be understanding of what the required task involves and sufficient memory to keep this in mind during the activity. It could be dangerous should a person be easily distracted by noise or movements within the room. A good level of concentration and ability to remain on task are essential. Concentration can be affected by motivation, and a person who is interested in the task and has aspirations to succeed is likely to have the necessary levels of motivation.

Scissors activities require a multitude of skills beginning with sensory input which is then perceived or made sense of. Perception leads to motor planning and subsequent motor output, all of which take place in the presence of memory, concentration, motivation and the ability to remain on task.

CHAPTER 3

Conditions that may delay or preclude the acquisition of scissors skills

There are many medical conditions that will make the use of scissors slow, uncomfortable, painful or require continuous conscious effort. Such conditions may be physical, cognitive or behavioural. In some conditions the use of scissors is not practical or a reasonable expectation. For others, attempts to use scissors could be definitely dangerous to the proposed user and/or other people.

Should the completed scissors project not come up to the expectations of the creator there will be disappointment and frustration. This will be true whether the person is a child or an adult. Expertise will be required to ascertain whether the degree of failure with the project is due to a physical, cognitive or behavioural condition that makes the project unsuitable for that person to attempt, or that the person has not had the opportunity to learn and develop the requisite skills.

In order to ascertain and classify problems that may be present or develop when using scissors, various conditions, and the symptoms that occur in them, will be discussed. It is often most relevant to consider the prevailing symptoms rather than the underlying condition or conditions, as particular symptoms may be more pertinent than the actual condition or syndrome.

Conditions may be classified as follows:

*   Congenital conditions: these are conditions that develop in the perinatal period, *in utero*, during birth or shortly after birth.
*   Acquired conditions: these are conditions that are acquired after birth, during childhood, adolescence or in adult life.

Conditions may also be divided into those that affect the senses, those that affect perception, cognition or behaviour and those that affect movement.

Sensory problems

The senses provide information about ourselves and our environment that is needed for any action, response or motor effect we make. The senses include vision or eyesight, hearing, taste, smell, touch and proprioception. It follows that any difficulty with the use of any of the senses will result in some loss of perception that could also lead to changes in motor response.

Visual acuity

Being able to see clearly the material that is to be cut is important both for the execution of the task and for safety. Visual acuity is the capacity for seeing the details of an object clearly. Therefore the visual acuity of the person doing the task must be known to the person setting up the scissors task.

Visual fields

A visual field is the space visible with eyes in a particular position. There are various conditions in which visual fields may be limited so care must be taken to ensure that any limitation is known. Limitation of visual fields may result in certain areas of vision being ignored, although many people adjust to the deficit by changes in head posture. Impairment of visual fields may be congenital or acquired, in conditions such as hemiplegia and head injury respectively.

Tunnel vision

In this condition, vision is limited to the central part of the visual field. It has serious effects on vision in both daily living activities and specific tasks. It can occur in glaucoma, where there is increased pressure within the eye, and retinitis pigmentosa, where there is deterioration of the retina at the back of the eye. It will be necessary to adjust the head position in order to see to the left or right, or superior or inferior visual areas.

Peripheral vision

Peripheral vision results from stimulation of the retina outside the fovea or macular region. In practice this means that vision is restricted to the periphery of normal visual fields. There is no central vision, which is normally used where hand–eye coordination is required. The head may be held in unusual positions so that the best use may be made of the peripheral vision.

Colour blindness

This term is often used to describe all forms of mild or severe colour vision deficiency. These problems are more prevalent in males than females. It is often referred to as 'defective colour vision'. Some people find very pale shades difficult to differentiate, others have difficulty with pink/orange or blue/green discrimination. Unless it is severe, colour vision deficiency may pass unnoticed. It is important that where colours are used they are such that the person with defective colour vision can appreciate them.

Nystagmus

This is a regular, repetitive, involuntary movement of the eye. The direction of the involuntary movement may be vertical, horizontal or diagonal. People with nystagmus often discover for themselves the head position in which the nystagmus is least troublesome. This may result in unusual head posture. For some people there may not be a position in which constant clear vision may be obtained.

Diplopia

In this condition a single object is seen as two objects rather than one object. This is because the images are not stimulating corresponding similar areas of the retina. The condition may be congenital or acquired later in life, usually due to trauma or brain surgery. Often people become used to their diplopia and learn to appreciate which is the 'real' image.

Myopia or short-sightedness

Myopia is a refractive condition in which distant objects are focused in front of the retina causing blurring of distance vision. Unless the condition is very severe it will not affect close work.

Hypermetropia or long-sightedness

This is a refractive condition in which distant objects are focused behind the retina causing blurring of vision. Usually the condition is corrected with glasses. It is important to be aware of the need for glasses especially for close work such as using scissors.

Presbyopia

This is a refractive condition of the eye in which accommodation becomes insufficient for satisfactory near vision. It usually begins to be apparent in the fifth decade of life. It is usually corrected by the use of glasses. Many older people choose to wear bifocal or varifocal lenses which will have the near vision element at the bottom of each lens. Care should be taken to ensure that the glasses fit well so that the correct part of the lens is used for close work.

Glaucoma

Glaucoma is a disease in which there is increased or unstable pressure within the eye. It requires treatment to prevent deterioration of the eye. According to the type of glaucoma, it can have various effects on vision. When teaching scissors skills, the effects of glaucoma should always be verified.

Cataract

Cataract is a visual impairment caused by loss of transparency of the lens of the eye. The degree of opacity of the lens varies according to the severity of the cataract and is usually progressive over time. It may be the result of trauma or disease, such as diabetes. Occasionally children are born with congenital cataracts. It is often possible to remove the cataracts which can result in dramatic improvement in the clarity of vision.

Tactile sensation

Sensitivity to touch, particularly in the hands, affects ability to perform motor skills. How objects are held, the amount of pressure exerted in the grip, is in part dependent on how they feel. For example an object which feels soft will be held with less pressure than one which feels hard or slippery. Numbness or partial numbness (paraesthesia) will affect fine motor skills such as using scissors. It will affect the delicacy of touch needed to hold paper without crumpling or damaging it in some other way. Loss of some of the sensitivity to touch may result in the person needing to monitor visually how the hands are used.

Pain

A small proportion of the population has impaired appreciation of pain and is unaware when they have caused themselves injury. Examples of such conditions are spina bifida and paraplegia. It is particularly important that people with such conditions work at a table or before a work surface to remove the danger of self-injury with the scissors, for in these conditions tactile sensation in the lower limbs may be impaired or absent.

Specialized nerves are concerned with the sensation of pain. A small percentage of the population has imperfect appreciation of pain as a symptom in the absence of any other neurological problems. A very small proportion of the population has complete absence of pain appreciation. Pain is a warning that something is amiss either internally or on the surface of the body. We have all, at some time, had sore fingers caused by using scissors to cut very tough material. People who do not have these warning signals, or have impaired signals, may cause themselves injury. One should choose suitable scissors and tasks for such people, and be aware of the possibility of skin or deeper tissue damage.

Proprioception

This is the appreciation of posture, balance and position of self by means of receptors, called proprioceptors, within muscles, joints and tendons, and the vestibular apparatus of the inner ear. People who have problems with proprioception may have difficulty with sitting balance and appreciating the position of body parts without resorting to visual clues. Poor proprioceptive skills are significant if they affect the hands and fingers when their position may not be perceived without visual monitoring.

Hearing

Although not directly connected to scissors skills, hearing can have some relevance to the task. When teaching, care should be taken that the person with impaired hearing has understood instructions. It may be that the person needs to watch the face of the speaker thus removing visual attention from the cutting process. It may be wise, particularly with children, to ensure that the closed scissors are placed on the table or work surface while instructions are given. The speaker's face should be in a good light especially where lip reading will take place. It may be advisable to provide verbal instructions and demonstrations separately so that the person with impaired hearing can watch the lips in the first instance and secondly give full attention to the demonstration.

Perception

The ability to process, organize and interpret sensory information from stimuli both within and outside the body is called perception. Should this ability be impaired, as the result of congenital problems or acquired ones, there is likely to be difficulty with many life activities as well as skilled tasks. Children who have developmental coordination disorder (DCD), dyspraxia or other coordination difficulties, and adults who have suffered a stroke, particularly one affecting the right side of the brain, should be assessed to ascertain if a perceptual deficit is one of the reasons for their difficulties. Other conditions in which there may be perceptual difficulties include head injuries or brain surgery, depending on the areas of the brain which are involved.

Body image

The basis of perception is appreciation of one's own body image. We all have an internal perception of our own size, shape and configuration. This is a constant, although unconscious, ability.

Spatial problems

Closely allied to this basic perception is that of our own position in space and relationships to other objects and people in space. We 'know' the position of ourselves at all times without the need for visual or manual reference to body parts. An everyday example of these skills is the process required to seat oneself in a chair. Without conscious thought the body is aligned with the chair, the body is lowered and the buttocks and thighs are placed on the seat of the chair. There is usually no difficulty with assessing the depth of the chair seat or the movements necessary to achieve a seated position. Similarly, standing up after being seated on a chair is an equally complex skill, yet it is accomplished without conscious thought, even from a chair which is unfamiliar.

The appreciation of position in space and spatial relationships of self and objects are important in all hand skills. In particular, with scissors activities, the appreciation of the relationships of the hands to the scissors, of the hands to the material being cut, and of the blades of the scissors to the material which is being cut, is vital. People who have difficulties in this area may find using scissors very difficult.

Figure/background problems

The ability to discriminate between foreground and background at both a fine and a gross level is important in most life skills. It can be applied to most of the senses. In a classroom situation there may be a number of noises such as chair legs being scraped on the floor, the pages of books being flipped through, coughs and chattering. Despite these extraneous noises, most children will be able to concentrate on what their neighbour is telling them. Only those with difficulty with figure/background discrimination will be distracted by the other noises in the room. A further example is that of older people with a small degree of hearing loss, who can hear adequately when having a personal conversation with one other person, but have difficulty hearing the person who is speaking to them when several people in their group are speaking simultaneously. These auditory problems could be significant when verbal instructions are being given about scissors skills.

Figure/background difficulties of a visual nature are often more significant to scissors skills. Should the material which is to be cut have a patterned background, the line upon which the scissors should cut may be difficult to distinguish from the pattern. If the material being cut is of a similar colour to the background against which it is being held, such as the table or work surface, it may be difficult to distinguish one from the other.

Attention deficit disorder (ADD)

Some people with ADD have problems only with maintaining attention; others also have hyperactivity, when the condition is described as attention deficit hyperactivity disorder (ADHD). These conditions are usually associated with children although remnants of the conditions may be observed in adolescents and adults. There is a particularly short concentration span which may vary according to the activity and circumstances in which it is undertaken. People with ADD or ADHD are usually easily distracted and impulsive. ADD and ADHD can occur with other conditions such as cerebral palsy, dyspraxia and Asperger's syndrome. Clearly, close supervision will be required when scissors are being used.

Epilepsy

Care should be taken when people who suffer from epilepsy are using scissors. Many people are aware of an impending seizure and will take safety precautions themselves. It is important to know details of the type, severity and expected frequency of seizures. Some people have momentary 'absences' and will be unaware of any instructions given during them. Other people have full-blown seizures where there is loss of consciousness; it is during these times that holding scissors could become hazardous. Seizures are usually well controlled in most people.

Motor activity

There are many symptoms and characteristics which affect movement or motor activity. Before movement can take place there must be planning or organization of movement at a cerebral level, usually called motor planning. Following this, the actual movement takes place.

Motor planning

This is the planning and organization of movement at a cerebral level which usually takes place without conscious effort. Difficulty in this area is known as dyspraxia, while the complete inability to plan or organize motor tasks is apraxia. Children are most often described as dyspraxic and usually demonstrate some improvement with maturity and treatment. Adults may develop some areas of apraxia following a cerebrovascular accident or stroke.

Difficulty with planning motor activity has serious effects on motor skills. Children with the condition take longer than usual to master skills and some may continue to have a degree of difficulty. Such difficulties resolve for some people but for others they continue into adult life. With the passage of time those who continue to have difficulties may find ways round them, choosing slip-on shoes, for instance, rather than those with laces to fasten, or using word processing rather than writing with a pen. Adults can lose skills at which they were previously adept following stroke or other cerebral accidents. Scissors skill is one such activity which may be affected.

Motor problems

There are a number of categories of symptom which can affect motor activity.

- Neurological symptoms result from functions and dysfunctions of a part or parts of the nervous system.
- Physical limitation of movement may be caused by joint abnormality or dysfunction, swelling or pain.
- Trauma to nerves, bones, muscles or soft tissue may temporarily or permanently affect movement.
- Congenital malformations of any body tissue may affect movement.

Neurological symptoms

Abnormalities of the central nervous system can have profound effects on the quality of movement. There may be lack of control of movement, limitation of movement, lack of power or extraneous movement preventing function. Function may be so greatly affected that the safe use of scissors is precluded.

Ataxia

This is a symptom which occurs in some types of cerebral palsy and other conditions such as acquired head injury. It is characterized by a coarse tremor which affects the head, trunk and limbs. For many affected people hand function will be so poor that activities such as using scissors will not be realistic and, indeed, for the most severely affected, may be dangerous.

Friedrich's ataxia is a progressive disease characterized by increasing ataxia, nystagmus and kyphoscoliosis. It manifests itself in childhood with such symptoms as 'clumsiness' or incoordination, and initially may be treated as such. Hand function will become increasingly impaired and overall ataxia will impair hand–eye coordination.

Athetosis

In athetosis, there are characteristic involuntary slow writhing movements and, sometimes, quick jerky movements which are called chorea. The condition is usually apparent during the first few months of life when there is marked developmental delay and retention of infant reflexes after the age at which they have disappeared in the average child. The symptoms persist throughout life.

Hemiplegia

Most strokes or cerebrovascular accidents result in some degree of hemiplegia, paralysis or partial paralysis of the left or right side of the body. Most strokes occur in people of mature years, although younger people do sometimes suffer one or more strokes. Occasionally very young children become hemiplegic. The most common type of hemiplegia in children is congenital, that is, present at birth or occurring very shortly afterwards. Usually the arm proves to be more severely affected than the leg. The effect is most significant when hemiplegia affects what is or would have been the preferred or dominant hand. Prolonged treatment programmes reduce the residual effects of both congenital and acquired hemiplegia.

With regard to using scissors, both hands are used, one to manipulate the scissors and the other to hold the material being cut. There may be difficulty holding the material cut in the hemiplegic hand because of increased muscle tone in that hand. The muscle tone is often increased when the other hand is in continuous use, as when using the reciprocal movement of opening and closing scissors. This increase of muscle tone results in contraction of the flexor muscles of the hand and often causes spoiling of the material being held.

Diplegia

Diplegia occurs in one of the earliest types of cerebral palsy to be described in the middle of the 19th century by Dr William Little. Occasionally it is still referred to as Little's disease. It is characterized by increased tone on the hamstring and adductor muscles of the legs which can cause problems with sitting, walking and balance. The development of ankle, knee and hip contractions is common though physiotherapy programmes help to prevent the development and reduce the severity of contractions. Seating will need careful consideration in order to minimize the development of contractions and to optimize sitting balance. Frequently slight difficulty with coordination and organization of movement patterns occurs in the upper limb, which will, of course, have an effect on all fine hand skills.

Tremor

Consideration of tremor, both normal and abnormal, is apposite to the acquisition of efficient scissors skills.

> *Each of us has a normal physiological tremor which is almost imperceptible to the naked eye. The frequency of the oscillations of physiological tremor varies with age from 6 cycles per second before 9 years to 10 cycles per second at 16 years, the frequency begins to decline after 40 years until it has returned to 6 cycles per second at 70 years. (Fahn 1972)*

Tremor may make fine hand skills difficult and, in severe cases, hand skills such as drawing, handwriting and using scissors may be so unsatisfactory and the results so poor that alternative methods such as word processing and the use of a paper trimmer will be advisable.

Dystonia

This term describes the symptom of slow writhing movements which can affect some or all muscle groups. There are a number of syndromes in which dystonia occurs including dystonia musculorum deformans.

Poor muscle power

Muscle weakness, or lack of power, is a symptom of many conditions including the dystrophies and atrophies. Some of these diseases are apparent at birth and are severe and life threatening; others are manifested later in childhood or early adult life.

- Duchenne muscular dystrophy is inherited through the mother and manifested in male children. It is cruelly progressive and usually a wheelchair is needed by the time the boy reaches the early teenage years and hand function becomes progressively more impaired.
- Becker muscular dystrophy is another condition which affects males. It is less severe than Duchenne type and its progression is slower.
- Limb girdle dystrophy affects both males and females. The rate of progression is variable but usually slow.
- Spinal muscular atrophy occurs in several forms. The main feature, in addition to muscle weakness, is contractures around joints.

Multiple sclerosis

Multiple sclerosis (MS), previously known as disseminated sclerosis, is a chronic disease in which degeneration of the white matter of the brain and spinal cord leads to progressive weakness and disability. The myelin covering nerve fibres is patchily destroyed, the axons become thin and sometimes disappear. These patches become sclerotic and result in the destruction and loss of conductivity of the nerve fibre. The disease usually becomes apparent between the ages of 20 and 40 years, and is slightly more common in women than men. There are usually remissions and relapses but it is difficult to predict the course the disease will take. Hand activity may be affected to greater or lesser degrees, and help with function will be needed on an individual basis. This will also vary according to the stage of the disease and relapses and remissions (Turner 1996).

Limitation of movement

Movement may be limited by a number of symptoms including inflammation, swelling, pain and scar tissue.

Arthritis

There are many types of arthritis which affect both children and adults.

Juvenile chronic arthritis (JCA) is not a single disease but a group of conditions which affect the joints of children and young people. The definition of JCA is that there must have been an arthritis of at least 3 months' duration, starting before the 16th birthday, with the exclusion of other diseases that could mimic the condition (Craft 1985). It may affect a small number of joints (pauciarticular) or many joints (poliarticular). There may be only one episode of disease or it may persist and fluctuate throughout childhood. During episodes of acute illness, hand skills, such as the use of scissors, will be out of the question. This will also apply to adult forms of rheumatoid arthritis.

At times when the arthritis has waned it is important to take measures to protect all the joints which have been affected. Undue pressure should not be exerted on them and sustained positions should be avoided. Special care will be required in the choice of scissors and how they are used. Some people will be prescribed orthoses or splints to maintain the wrist and joints of the hand in an optimum position and to avoid the possibility of the development of contractures. Splints may be worn only at night, or additional working splints may be worn during the day to maintain the wrist in a position midway between flexion and extension, or in a degree of wrist extension. The latter usually have a narrow strip of splinting material which lies in the cleft between the thumb and index finger, which could, for some people, cause discomfort when using scissors.

Scleroderma

This is a condition in which there are flexion deformities with tight, waxy skin. It may begin to develop in the hands and face and spread to other parts of the body. Manual activities are usually particularly affected as the disease progresses and the use of scissors may not be possible.

Morquio syndrome

Morquio syndrome is one of the disorders of metabolism of complex sugars known as mucopolysaccharidoses (MPS). There is poor growth and adult height is very much below average. There is laxity of the ligaments which support joints, and this is significant to all motor activity. One of most serious abnormalities is instability of the atlantoaxial joint. Various types of the syndrome have been described with differing degrees of severity (Penso 1992). Eventually hand function is likely to be impaired.

Burns and other injuries

During the acute stages of these injuries, hand activities are likely to be inappropriate. During the recovery stages, when scar tissue and contractures are a possibility, activities such as the use of scissors may need to be limited and adapted to suit each type of limitation.

Congenital conditions

Arthrogryposis

This is a congenital disorder of the connective tissue which encapsulates joints. It results in varying degrees of limitation of movement. Joints may be fixed in flexion, extension or in more complex abnormal positions. For example, the wrist may be fixed in flexion and internal rotation. If this wrist position is combined with the elbow and shoulder being fixed in abnormal positions, hand function will be seriously impaired. Sometimes surgery is advised to move one or more of the joints into a more functional position. The condition may occur on its own or in combination with other conditions, such as spinal muscular atrophy or partial limb deficiency.

Osteogenesis imperfecta

This congenital condition is more commonly described as 'brittle bones'. A seemingly trivial fall, or even an everyday movement, can result in a fracture which proves difficult to heal. There is poor growth resulting in small stature and deformity in some people. Life experiences may be limited because of the ever present danger of fractures. Advice should be taken regarding the suitability of scissors activities, and, even when judged to be appropriate, they should be planned with care.

Achondroplasia

There are several types of achondroplasia and a number of related syndromes (Jones 1988). The epiphyses of the long bones unite at an earlier stage of development than normal, thus preventing further growth of the long bones resulting in the characteristic short limbs. In some types of achondroplasia there is arthritic pain which can become severe. The hands are exceptionally broad with very short fingers; these characteristics impede hand function and repetitive finger movements may become painful. Scissors will need to be specially chosen to suit the dimensions of the hand.

Syndactylism

Syndactylism is a congenital condition. In mild cases, there is webbing of the fingers and/or toes. The degree of resulting difficulty with hand function will depend on the severity of the webbing. When the condition is severe there is fusion of two or more digits and sometimes of the nails too. Sometimes it is possible surgically to separate two or more digits. For finger separation to be feasible, each fused finger must have its own bone structure. Syndactylism is one of the symptoms which occurs in Apert's syndrome.

Upper limb deficiency

There are a number of rare syndromes in which there is partial or complete upper limb deficiency. Sometimes only one or more digits are absent. These deficiencies are present at birth. Fingers or limbs may also be lost as the result of a traumatic accident or injury. Hand activities will be limited according to the degree of loss, and adaptations to equipment will be needed on an individual basis. It is usually more effective to make adaptations to facilitate activities for those who have a mechanical deficit, such as absent digits, than for those who have neurological dysfunction.

CHAPTER 4

Sitting and other positions in which scissors may be used

Most people sit when they are using scissors. There are exceptions, such as when kitchen scissors are used to joint a chicken or snip herbs when the best position will usually be standing at a work surface. For children, however, it is best to insist on a stable sitting position for reasons of safety, concentration and application to the task.

Chairs

As discussed in Chapter 2, in order to attain optimum hand function, the trunk and arms must have stability. This is normally effected by having a chair such that the depth of the seat supports the thighs. The chair should not be so deep that its front edge presses into the back of the knees, which would be uncomfortable and could cause pressure on nerves or impede blood flow to some degree. The height of the chair seat from the floor should be such that the feet are plantigrade on the floor and the knee joints form a right angle (Figure 4.1).

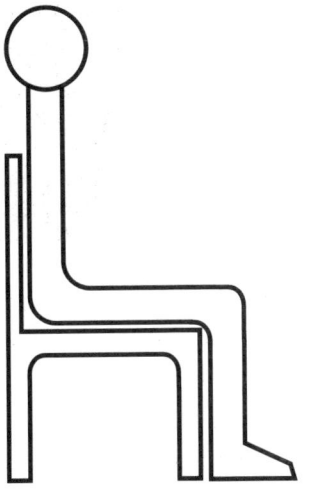

Figure 4.1 Diagrammatic representation of a good basic sitting position on a chair of the correct height from the floor so that the feet are plantigrade and the thighs are supported by the depth of the chair seat.

(First appeared in Penso DE (1993) Perceptuo-motor Difficulties: theory and strategies to help children, adolescents and adults. Chapman & Hall. Reproduced by permission of Nelson Thornes Ltd.)

A chair which is inappropriately large or disproportionate to the person sitting on it will become uncomfortable if it is used for all but the briefest period. It will promote a poor posture and reduce trunk stability (Figures 4.2 and 4.3). The person will need to give attention to sitting balance rather than to the task being undertaken. Those with attention deficit disorder will have difficulty sitting still.

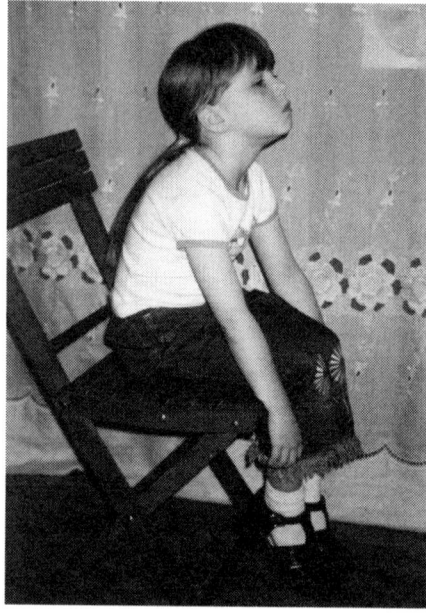

Figure 4.3 Alice is sitting comfortably on a chair which is of the correct dimensions for her. In this position she would be able to undertake hand activities successfully. Her feet are plantigrade, her thighs supported and the chair back is appropriate for her.

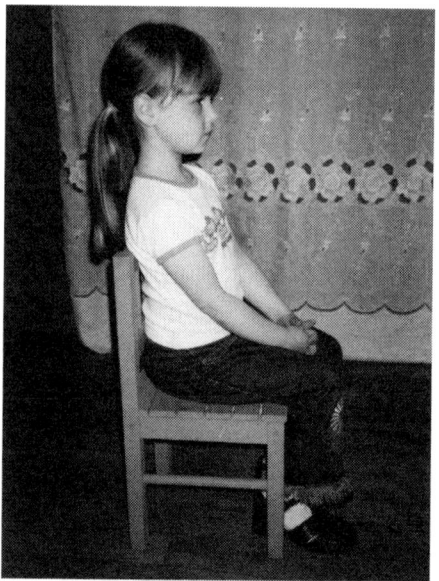

Figure 4.2 It is obvious that Alice is uncomfortable and unstable sitting on this chair which is too high, too deep from back to front and the chair back is at an inappropriate angle.

It is possible to adjust the height of chair seats from the floor for both children and adults, to ensure that the chair is of the correct height. This may be achieved using chair raisers (Figure 4.4).

A step attached to the front of a chair will allow children of comparatively short stature to use chairs of a similar height to their peers so that they may be

(a)

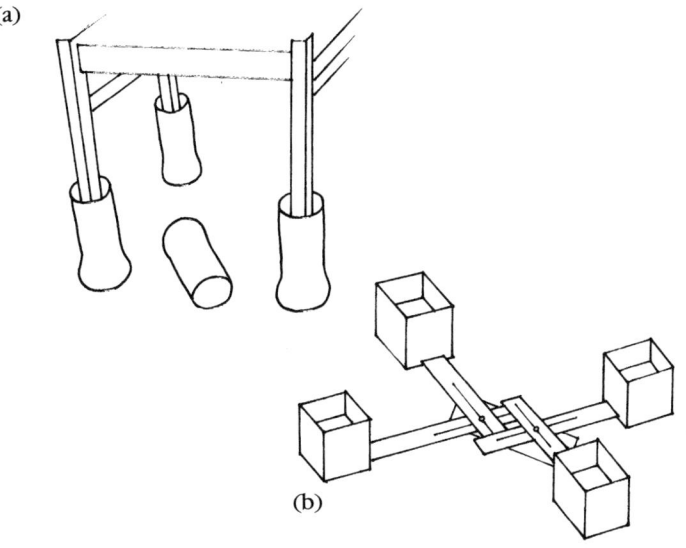

(b)

Figure 4.4 a. Plastic chair raisers, fluted on the internal surface to hold the chair legs securely.

b. Wooden chair raisers with adjustable bars which enable the raisers to be fitted to chairs of various dimensions.

(First appeared in Penso DE (1990) Keyboard, Graphic and Handwriting Skills: helping people with motor disabilities. Chapman & Hall. Reproduced by permission of Nelson Thornes Ltd.)

appropriately seated at the same table as their group (Figure 4.5). For children who have difficulty keeping their feet still, a non-slip surface added to the step is useful. For children who have athetosis or other similar neurological problems, wool carpet will reduce the noise of feet constantly moving. Wool carpet is suggested rather than synthetic carpet because the former is less slippery.

(a)

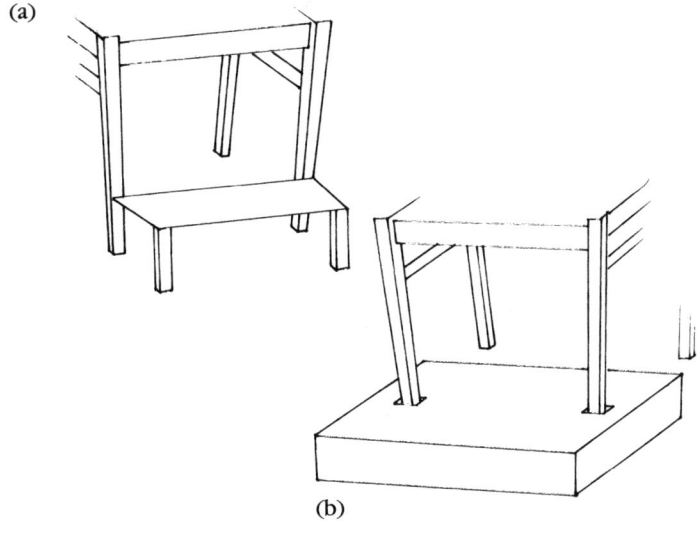

(b)

Figure 4.5 a. A home-made foot rest which is attached to the front of the chair.

b. A quickly made foot rest that uses a wooden box of suitable height in which two holes are cut to accommodate the front legs of the chair.

(First appeared in Penso DE (1990) Keyboard, Graphic and Handwriting Skills: helping people with motor disabilities. Chapman & Hall. Reproduced by permission of Nelson Thornes Ltd.)

Some people may feel more secure and indeed be able to sustain a stable position more easily if their chair has sides or arms. The sides of the chair should not hamper hand function, nor should they prevent the chair being drawn up to the table. Arms or sides on the chair may also form a rest on which the elbows may be placed, whilst keeping the upper arms close to the body, to increase stability of the upper limbs.

For people who have difficulty sitting still, a piece of non-slip material, such as Dycem®, may reduce unnecessary movements. Care should be taken, however, for some people cannot tolerate sitting on a completely non-slip surface.

Work surfaces

The table or work surface should be sufficiently high for the legs to fit comfortably underneath it without the knees pressing against the under surface. It should be of such a height that the forearms with elbows flexed may comfortably rest upon it. For small children and those with a particularly short trunk, it is better if the table does not have a stretcher between the legs. A deep stretcher or bar between the table legs and the table top will increase the depth of the table top and will cause the person who sits up to the table to sit at a lower level in order to avoid the stretcher. Thus the level of the top of the table will be inappropriately high on the body of the person.

For people who have a short trunk, who have shorter than average arms or who have a large or protruding abdomen, a table with a semi-circular cut out on the edge to which they will be sitting will increase comfort and allow the arms or elbows to rest on the table. Because the table will partly encircle the body it will increase trunk stability.

The colour of the worktop can also help or impede scissors skills. Those with visual difficulties will benefit from a high degree of contrast between the top of the work surface and the materials being used. A plain rather than patterned surface is preferable for those who are easily distracted, those with visual difficulties and those who have problems with figure/background discrimination.

The texture of the worktop should also be considered. Those who have difficulty moving objects on the work surface or who have little muscle power will benefit from a surface with little friction; a smooth surface. Conversely those who have instability such as ataxia, dystonia or athetosis, will benefit from a work surface which provides friction; a surface which has some texture. Dycem® provides an ideal non-slip surface, which may be of particular benefit for those who have to manipulate the scissors and control the material being cut with the heel or side of the same hand.

Some people cope better with a sloping surface, the optimum degree of which can be ascertained by a little experimentation. The slope can help both the position of the forearms and vision. Light falls on a sloping surface at a different angle to a horizontal one and this can benefit some people with visual problems.

There are situations for both children and adults when a person's best hand function is attained when standing or leaning against a high level surface. This is acceptable when the person has stability in a standing position, but not appropriate where there is instability due to ataxia, spasticity or another neurological or mechanical problem. Instead of standing, it may be possible to use a higher chair than is usual so that the trunk is high in relation to the table. This will allow the elbows, or, for some people, the forearms, to be rested on the work surface. In this position it will be possible to bear weight through the upper arms, thus increasing stability. For some people with severe problems with trunk control, a standing box, standing frame or even a prone board may be used (Figure 4.6). Often such

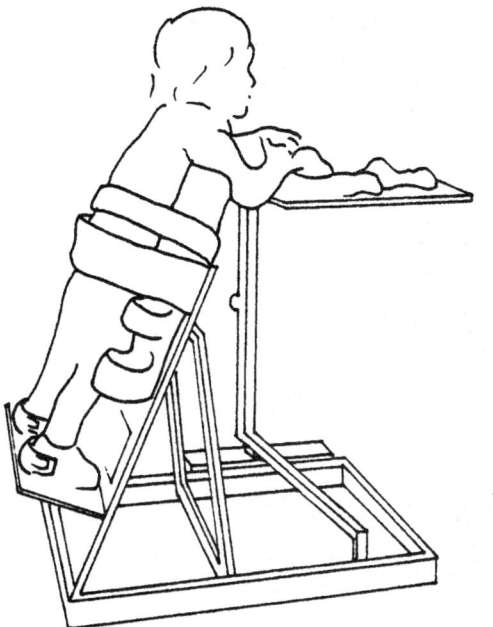

Figure 4.6 One version of an adjustable standing frame. There is a variety of models available to suit the various needs of both children and adults.

(First appeared in Penso DE (1990) Keyboard, Graphic and Handwriting Skills: helping people with motor disabilities. Chapman & Hall. Reproduced by permission of Nelson Thornes Ltd.)

people will already have had such a piece of equipment prescribed. It is important that they are carefully placed in such pieces of equipment so that they are positioned safely, with special attention given to joint and limb position.

Safety considerations

Everyone is aware that scissors, if they are misused, can be very dangerous both to the user and other people. The following points should be borne in mind whenever scissors are being used. Some of the points will be more appropriate to children and others to all people.

- Whenever a person is walking from one place to another with scissors in their hands, the scissors should be held with the blades closed and enclosed within a flexed hand. The scissors are then of no danger to the person carrying them or to other people.
- When scissors are being given to another person the blades should always be carried in a closed hand so that the handles of the scissors are given to the other person (Figure 4.7).

Figure 4.7 Joanna is holding a pair of closed scissors safely in preparation either to hand them to another person or to walk whilst holding them.

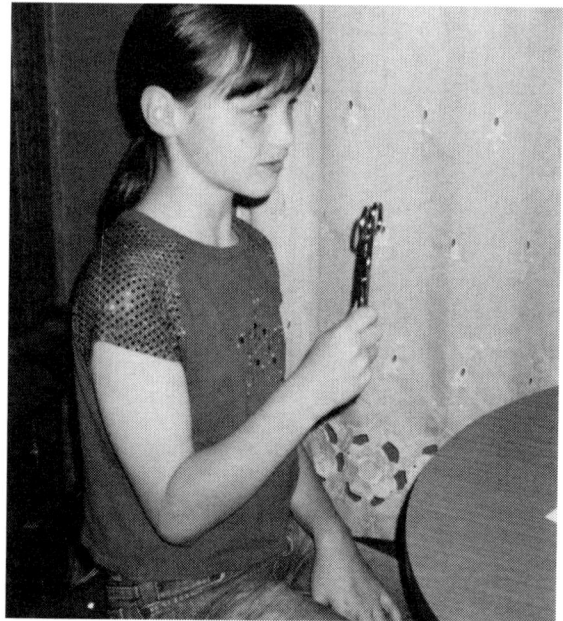

- The person using the scissors should always be in a stable position. This is most usually a sitting position. An exception to this would be a person using scissors to cut out the pieces of material prior to making a garment. In such a situation it is important to ensure that passage is not impeded around the table on which the material is arranged. This is particularly important where there is any unsteadiness, as is a non-slip floor surface.
- Scissors should be used with the blades pointing away from the person using them. This is almost always the best position in which to hold scissors.
- Scissors should only be used for their intended purpose. One blade with the scissors in an open position should not be used for scoring lines on paper, card or other materials. The point of scissor blades should not be used for making holes in any kind of material.

The safe use of scissors cannot be too strongly emphasized, but at the same time care should be taken not to make users of scissors over-sensitive to the possible dangers. An occupational therapist who was working in a psychiatric hospital was referred a young woman in her twenties who had a phobia for 'points' of scissors and knives. She suffered from mild cerebral palsy which limited her hand function to some extent. She had been conditioned into her phobic state by her anxious, over-protective mother who constantly warned her to take care every time she picked up a pointed or sharp object. Her occupational therapist devised a carefully graded desensitization programme and, over a period of time, she made good progress and was able to convince her mother that she could handle scissors safely.

Safety is important, but the necessary precautions must be presented in a positive manner.

CHAPTER 5

Pre-scissors skills

Should there be problems with a child developing scissors skills, there are activities which can be used to encourage the underlying functions necessary for scissors to be used effectively. Parallel activities may also be used to help adults who have never acquired scissors skills. For children and adults who have lost previously acquired skills, because of injury or progressive disease, different approaches will be needed.

The types of activities which may be used to further the development of scissors skills are those which are directly concerned with hand function, those which are concerned with overall position and stability and those which are concerned with the necessary intellectual and behavioural abilities.

Activities to help hand function

Poking and pushing

Poking and pushing to make holes in Playdoh® or modelling clay (Plasticene®) with one or more fingers will help hand function. The resistance of the material used will vary according to the child's muscle power. Where appropriate, the resistance of the material may be increased commensurate with an increase in muscle power. Games may also be devised which involve pinching the material, perhaps to make models of animals such as hedgehogs complete with spines. In homes where there is baking, and particularly pastry making, children enjoy activities such as pinching the edges of pastry pies and pasties together.

Painting

Painting using whole hands helps with wrist extension and bearing weight through the arm. Finger painting using individual fingers draws attention to each finger and exerts pressure on each one. The painting can include dabbing with individual fingers as well as drawing enclosed shapes such as circles and squares which will encourage medial and lateral deviation at the metacarpophalangeal joint. Care should be taken, however, because some children do not enjoy having their hands soiled or sticky.

Finger games

Finger games may be used with young children and, in addition to drawing attention to the fingers, they are an excellent means of encouraging interaction with other people. A number of nursery rhymes lend themselves to finger games such as 'One two three four five, Once I caught a fish alive' and 'Tommy Thumb, Tommy Thumb, Where are you?'. Iona and Peter Opie have collected children's rhymes, many of which may be adapted to use with the fingers (Opie and Opie 1992). Older children will enjoy more sophisticated games which include finger activities, such as spinning tiny spinning tops and tiddlywinks. The Opies have made a comprehensive collection of children's games, some of which will provide inspiration for purposeful finger exercises (Opie and Opie 1997).

Squeezing and squashing

Squeezing and squashing to produce a sound holds a fascination for many children. Tiny metal 'clickers' are fun (although perhaps not for parents' ears!). Bubble wrap intended for packing parcels is great fun to pop between finger and thumb. It should always be used under close supervision because it is a plastic material which should be kept away from the mouth. The foil inners from wine boxes when semi-inflated are interesting to squeeze and squash. Again they should only be used under close supervision.

Finger puppets

Finger puppets encourage individual finger movements. Representations of people or animals, birds or fish may be drawn directly on to fingers with washable non-toxic pens. Depending on the age and ability of the child, activities may be graded from moving a particular finger on which a specific character is depicted, to allowing two or more characters to 'meet', thus encouraging opposition of fingers to the thumb or fingers to each other.

There are various types of finger puppet, from a simple tube of paper or thin card which is made to fit the ends of the fingers, to commercially available cloth puppets which fit the fingers. The latter are often sold in groups with a theme such as a fairy story, circus characters or farm animals. Such puppets can also be home-made. Puppets should always be introduced gently for some children are apprehensive of things which move seemingly without human intervention.

To encourage reciprocal movements of the index and ring fingers cardboard characters may be drawn omitting the legs. Two circles are cut out of the lower part of the body to accommodate the index and middle fingers which become the 'legs' of the puppet. The puppet is animated by reciprocal finger movements.

A dark coloured glove can have a 'face' sewn or glued on to each finger which will encourage individual finger movements. This is an activity more suitable for older children who are able to place their fingers in the fingers of the glove with minimum help.

Hand puppets

Hand puppets which need the thumb in one arm of the puppet and the little finger, or ring and little finger, in the other, with the remaining two or three fingers in the neck of the puppet encourage finger movements where the child is unable to monitor those fingers visually.

Computer keyboards

Computer keyboards can be excellent means of using individual fingers. The activity can be graded to suit the ability and interests of the user. Learning fingering for word processing is perhaps the best way to have consistent practice with purposeful use of each finger (Penso 1999).

Activities to help position and stability

Any fine motor activity is best accomplished when adopting the most stable sitting position possible. For some people, sitting may not be their best position and standing with arms supported and bearing weight through the upper arms may best facilitate hand function. For a few people a standing box with a work tray or a prone angle board with work tray will facilitate the most stable position. When using scissors the importance of a stable position cannot be too greatly emphasized.

It is good practice to encourage the optimum working position for all activities so that it is adopted spontaneously and, in particular, when undertaking scissors activities.

Activities to help intellectual and behavioural ability

Looking

Looking is imperative when undertaking scissors skills. Any activity which encourages visual concentration is helpful, such as reciprocal games of rolling a ball back and forth between two people, most usually the child concerned and an adult, the latter giving frequent reminders to watch the ball and be ready to hold the approaching ball. Any toy which has balls or marbles running along channels will encourage visual following, especially if there is also an element of noise. Very young children enjoy watching coloured bubbles rise in an illuminated tube. A bubble tube is expensive, but perhaps its cost can be justified when a number of people will benefit from it. With all these toys, adult supervision and encouragement is advised so that the child positively watches and does not just become mesmerized by the movements of the toy.

Concentration

Concentration is a problem for some children and adults. With all scissors activities, concentration on the task is important if the activity is to be successful as well as safe. Any activity can be used to encourage concentration and the length of the concentration span. Begin with very brief activity goals and stop immediately when that goal is reached. Do not be tempted to continue because the child or adult is 'doing well'. Stop on a high note of success, so that when the activity is next attempted the memory of past success will be uppermost in the mind, thus providing a good mental set for further periods of concentration.

Motivation

Motivation, or the desire to acquire scissors skills or undertake an activity, is very important. If motivation is not present, progress will not be made, no matter what the skill level is. Motivation evolves from success and, therefore, the task attempted must be at a level which ensures success. It is better to begin extremely simply with very small tasks, both with regards to amount of effort and amount of time needed to complete them. Thus it will be possible to demonstrate that success is possible. Where appropriate, showing a completed example of the task will often motivate the desire to attempt it. In a similar way as described in the section on concentration, stopping an activity once the goal has been reached will allow feelings of success to remain for future activities.

Motivation depends on realistic assessment of current abilities and fitting the activity exactly to those abilities, even if this requires progress to be in very small steps.

Activities to help children and adults to regain scissors skills

Remedial putty

Remedial putty may be used to encourage hand and individual finger movements. Its regular use will encourage the development of muscle power for many people. The putty is available in a number of strengths, which provide various degrees of resistance to hand and finger movement. Care is needed if it is used by over-enthusiastic children who pull it into thin strings; those strings can adhere to clothing. One colour should be used at a time, as different coloured putties placed next to each other will merge together and be almost impossible to separate.

Squashy balls

Kneading and squeezing squashy balls will encourage flexion and extension of the fingers and hand.

Finger exercises

Finger exercises can be used which encourage flexion and extension of each finger, and medial and lateral extension. Apposing each finger in turn to the thumb of the same hand approximates to the movements needed to use conventional scissors.

CHAPTER 6

Types of scissors and materials which may be cut

Before considering the style of scissors which would be best for a person to use, the hand, left or right, in which the scissors will be held should considered. It is very important that scissors are chosen to suit either the left or right hand in which they will be held. It has been estimated that between 87 and 90% of the population is right-handed (Paul 1997). It follows, therefore, that the majority of scissors which are manufactured are for right-handed use. Until recent years it was difficult to buy left-handed scissors but many types of scissors are now made to suit either left- or right-handed use.

Deciding on handedness

Most adults are well aware of the hand they prefer to use when cutting with scissors: only that preferred hand will feel comfortable and it will be the hand over which the person feels they have the most precise motor control. A number of adults will have suffered injury or disease which may prevent the preferred hand being used. With adequate practice and motivation many such people develop acceptable skills in what was the unpreferred hand. They will usually have to give more attention, motor planning and continuous concentration when using scissors and undertaking other fine motor tasks. Their performance may always be slower than previously when using the innately preferred hand.

There are some innately left-handed adults who, as children, were forced to use their right hand for cultural or other reasons. One still meets adults and the parents of some children who believe life will be easier if use of the right hand is encouraged. Those people, who have been forced to use their right hand, may consider themselves to be less than agile when undertaking fine motor skills; it may be worthwhile to experiment using the left hand and decide if its use would result in increased agility.

There are children whose first attempts to use scissors will be a two-handed activity with one hand operating each of the handles in the style of garden shears. With help, most children are able to manipulate scissors with one hand. At first it is a good idea to offer the closed scissors to the child in a mid-line position so that there is an absolutely free choice regarding the hand in which they will be used. A small number of children are late deciding which is their preferred hand. This may be a simple developmental problem which will resolve with maturation, or it may of a more complex nature. There may be conflict between the innately preferred hand and the hand which has the greatest agility, resulting in the child using one hand then reverting to using the other hand (Penso 1987; Bishop 1990). This could be the result of a very mild hemiplegia, dyspraxia or developmental coordination disorder.

Both children and adults may use a different hand for different fine motor activities (Barsley 1966). Several observers have noted that the more fine motor activities that are considered, the less well defined is hand preference. There could be an element of choosing one hand for precision activities and the other for those which require strength. The author has met several people who write with a pen held in one hand but prefer to use scissors held in the opposite hand.

Left- and right-handed scissors

Figure 6.1 shows a pair of left-handed scissors. The blades are arranged so that in use the blade which is on top does not obscure the line of cutting. In addition, when the correct scissors are chosen according to the hand in which they are held, as the blades come together in the action of cutting they will be drawn close to each other and thus make a good clean cut. Conversely, if scissors are used in the hand for which they are not intended, the upper blade will obscure the cutting line and, as the blades are closed in the action of cutting, they will tend to be drawn apart. Practical tests of these facts will illustrate them well. It is suggested that the reader tries using scissors which are designed for the opposite hand to which they use them and see how difficult it is to monitor the cutting line and to close the blades satisfactorily. In the case of large scissors, such as dressmaking shears, where the blades are longer and the superior edge is wider, using the correct scissors for the left or right hand is particularly important.

Large scissors also have handles which are shaped to fit comfortably round the thumb. Should a left-handed person attempt to use right-handed scissors, the curve

Figure 6.1 Early Learning Centre left-handed children's scissors. Note the left-handed configuration of the blades and compare them with the configuration of the blades on right-handed scissors. Notice also that the handles are plastic foam lined for comfort in use.

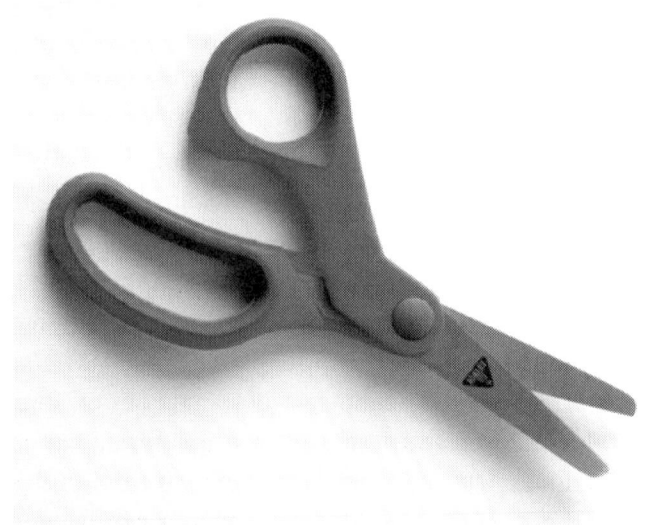

of the handle will make them uncomfortable to use as they will dig into the superior and lateral metacarpophalangeal joint. Some left-handed people who use right-handed scissors turn them upside down so that they are more comfortable round the thumb, but this does not remove the problem of the blades being wrongly aligned for them.

Today there should be no problem obtaining left-handed scissors from educational and therapeutic suppliers. They may need to be specially ordered when making a retail purchase. When buying sets of scissors for use in schools it should be remembered that, on average, at least 10% of the pupils in any class will require left-handed scissors. Where there is a number of children in a school who have developmental coordination disorder (DCD), dyspraxia or similar conditions, there is likely to be a larger proportion of children who are left-handed (Bishop 1990; Penso 1993). Some of these children will require special types of scissors in addition to their being for left-handed use.

There are many left-handed adults who have suffered discomfort when using scissors. These same people are likely to be dissatisfied with the quality and inaccuracy of their own cutting skills because they have never been introduced to scissors to suit their handedness. The more left-handed people who request left-handed scissors, the more shops are likely to stock them.

Choosing appropriate scissors for the person and the task

Scissors are available for almost any task for which it is possible to use them. It is preferable to keep scissors which are used for cutting paper for that task alone, for it is said that paper tends to blunt the blades. Similarly scissors which are used for cutting hair are best kept for that particular task. Dressmaking shears should only be used for cutting out fabric and a small pair of scissors should be available to cut thread. Because cutting thread uses only a minute part of the blade the scissors will become unevenly blunted and eventually this will render them unsuitable for cutting out fabric. In short, use the scissors which are intended for the task being undertaken.

Scissors for general use

Both scissors for children and for adults are now available with 'soft' lined foam handles which prevent any hard material, metal or plastic touching the skin. These scissors will provide greater comfort for those with thin skin of the hands, especially over joint areas.

Conventional, and some special, scissors are available with a self-opening spring mechanism which only requires movement to close the blades, not to open them (Figure 6.2). This mechanism is often helpful for people, particularly

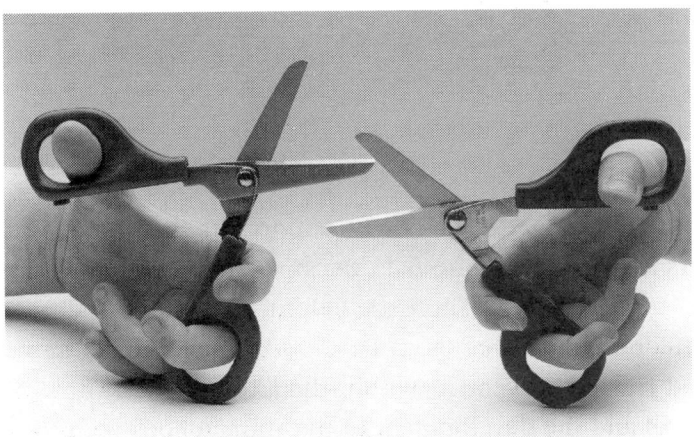

Figure 6.2 Peta self-opening scissors which are sprung to open when pressure is released. Because their default position is with the blades opened they are supplied with a guard, so that when not in use the blades are secured in the closed position.

children, who have difficulty with the repeated reciprocal movements required to activate conventional scissors. Many people who lack muscle power find them useful, as do people with cerebellar problems which prevent smooth reciprocal movements.

Self-opening scissors with a long loop handle which will comfortably accommodate the middle, ring and little fingers, with the index finger resting outside the loop, are helpful for people who have poor muscle power (Figure 6.3). This type of scissors allows all the fingers to be used to close the blades. They are also helpful for children who are more comfortable using all their fingers rather than just the index and middle fingers. Clearly they will be of great help to people who have fused fingers, such as occurs in Apert's syndrome. It is impossible for such people to use conventional scissors, which have handles designed to accommodate only one finger.

Figure 6.3 Peta self-opening scissors with a long loop handle to accommodate two or more fingers.

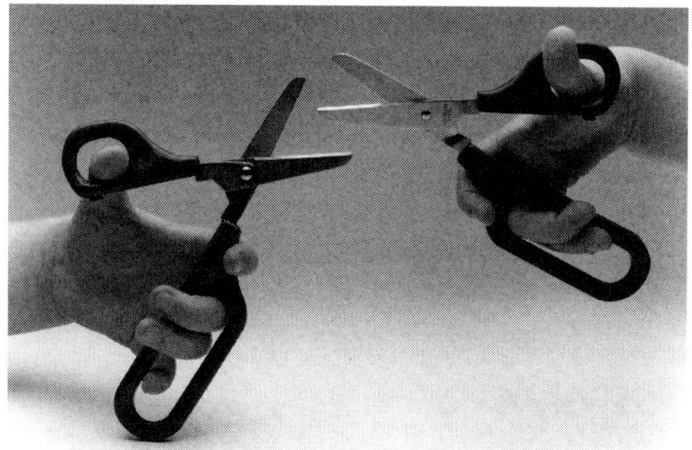

A number of manufacturers produce scissors with a loop, rather than handles, through which the fingers are placed (Figure 6.4). Because of the design of this type of scissors they must be self-opening. These are helpful for people of all ages with various problems. Children who have not yet developed precise finger movement find the whole-hand flexing movement within their capabilities. Thus the scissors are easier to control and the development of the spontaneous reciprocal hand movements, necessary to manipulate the scissors without visual monitoring

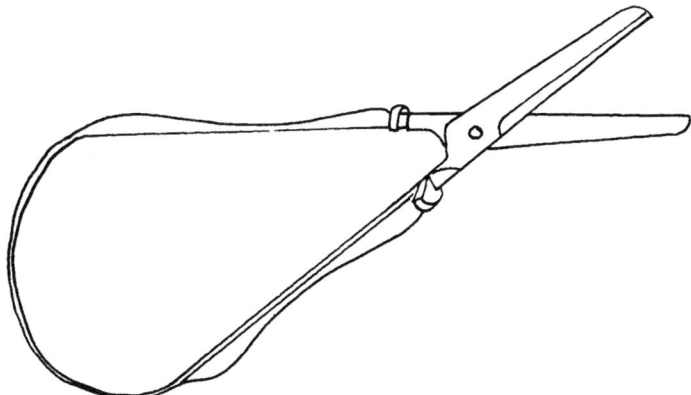

Figure 6.4 Whole-hand grip scissors which are self opening and remove the need for individual finger movements.

or conscious thought, is facilitated. Children are then able to concentrate on the cutting activity rather than the manipulation of the scissors. For the first time many children are delighted with their success with cutting and develop the motivation to continue with the activity and increase their skill level.

People with enlarged joints of the fingers may find that the handles of conventional scissors do not comfortably accommodate their fingers or thumb. Whole-hand grip scissors exert no pressure on these joints. They may be the only type of scissors which people with arthritis in the hands are able to use. However, anyone with arthritis, particularly in the acute stage, should be advised against using any scissors for prolonged periods, as this can cause discomfort, inflammation and intra-joint pressure, and holding joints in the same position for long periods is contraindicated.

Whole-hand grip scissors are available with blades in a variety of sizes from 30 mm to 75 mm. The smallest size is particularly useful for the small hands of children as well as for adults with small hands. They are useful for small, precise tasks, whilst the ones with longer blades can be used for longer straight cuts and, therefore, for different uses. Round-tipped scissors are safer for children to use. Those with pointed tips will be easier to use for tasks where small, very precise cuts are required.

Whole-hand grip scissors are available with a loop to accommodate the middle, ring and little fingers (Figure 6.5). This may be helpful when it is difficult to maintain flexion of the fingers to hold the handle or when the fingers tend to slip down the handle.

Figure 6.5 Whole hand grip scissors with a loop to accommodate the middle, ring and little fingers.

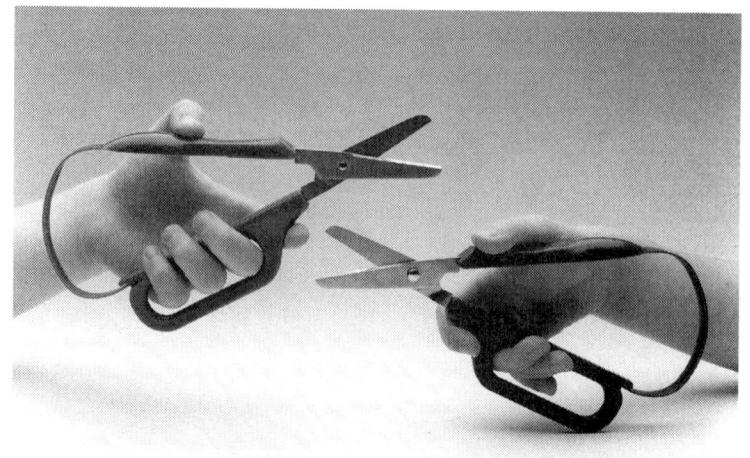

Small lightweight palmar grip scissors may help those with limited finger movement (Figure 6.6). As their name suggests, they fit into the palm of the hand and are activated by flexing the metacarpophalangeal joint. They have a spring action, so that release of the flexion movement results in the blades being opened. They are only suitable for small amounts of cutting, such as cutting thread or small pieces of paper. It is not possible to make long sweeping cuts with them. A serious disadvantage for all but steady hands is that the blades are very pointed and could easily pierce the skin.

Figure 6.6 Small palmar grip scissors which are suitable for small cutting tasks.

(First appeared in Penso DE (1990) Occupational Therapy for Children with Disabilities. Croom Helm Limited. Reproduced by permission of Nelson Thornes Ltd.)

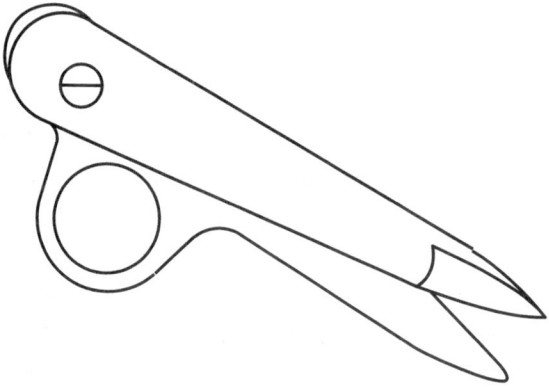

Training scissors are available mainly for use by children and a therapist or teacher. The scissors have double looped handles: the teacher or therapist uses those nearer to the blades, and the student uses the peripheral handles (Figure 6.7). This procedure can be used to help to develop the reciprocal movement necessary to cut with scissors. It will also help with concentration and help to steady the hand with a slight tremor. There may be instances where the child needs a very minimum of guidance and the loops used by the child and the therapist or teacher can be reversed.

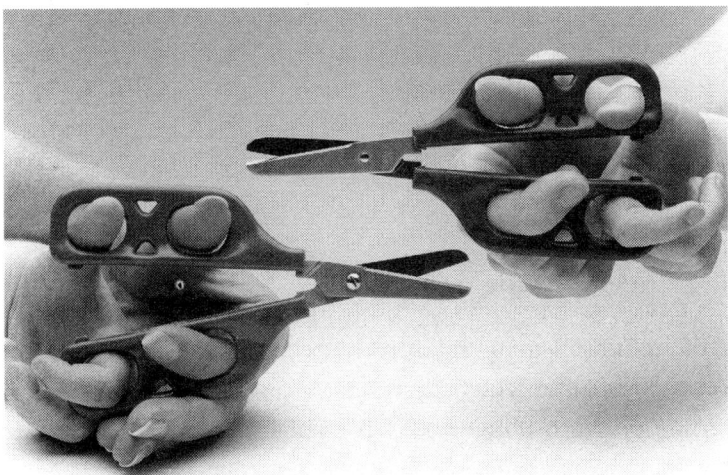

Figure 6.7 An example of training scissors with which both the student and the teacher or therapist may each hold one of the two pairs of loops of the scissors. They are useful to stimulate reciprocal opening and closing of the blades and other skills such as accurate cutting along a line.

Although not strictly scissors, a rolling paper cutter may help some people who would otherwise be unable to cut paper, thin card or film. The cutting part is concealed so that there is no danger of the user injuring herself. The cutting takes place by pulling the paper through the cutter (Figure 6.8).

Paper trimmers are a practical alternative for those whose hands are very unsteady. The cutting parts are completely concealed and so cannot damage the person using them. Although it is only possible to use paper trimmers for straight cuts, those cuts will be neat and accurate. A bar at the side of the paper trimmer allows the paper to be aligned at right angles to the cutting area, and a transparent bar, under which the paper is placed, allows it to be safely held in position whilst the cut is made. Paper trimmers are also useful for those who find cutting along a straight line difficult.

Figure 6.8 The rolling paper cutter is operated by pulling the paper through the cutter. The cutting edge is concealed so that it is safe to use. It will cut paper, card or film but not fabrics. It functions equally well in the right or left hand.

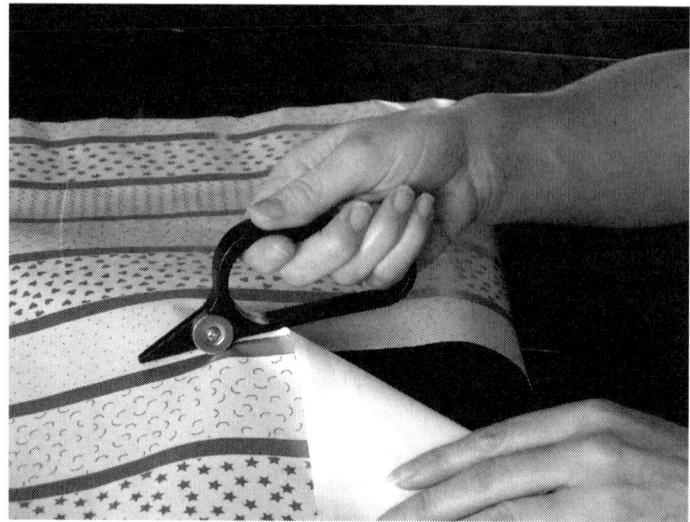

Equipment for cutting finger and toe nails

It is, of course, inadvisable to allow small children to try to cut their toe or finger nails. Simple nail scissors are available which have small curved blades which facilitate making a slightly rounded cut on finger nails. Toe nails should be cut straight across to prevent them ingrowing. Straight-edged toe nail cutters are available specifically to achieve this straight cut. Another type of toe nail cutter gives a long reach for those who have difficulty with bending to reach the toes (Figure 6.9). The long loop handle allows three fingers to be inserted, with the index finger used for extra control outside the handle. The blades are angled to give a good cutting position (Figure 6.9).

There are also ambidextrous nail scissors which adapt for either left- or right-handed use.

An alternative to nail scissors is the nail clipper, which is readily available in most chemists and department stores. Several sizes are made. They require a finger/thumb squeezing action to use them. Their advantage is that they may be carefully positioned before the cut is made with the hand supported on a firm surface for stability. A version is available which is mounted on a plastic base with non-slip feet (Figure 6.10). A large finger pad on the lever, which activates the cutting, allows more fingers to be used and requires downward pressure of the hand rather than the finer and more complex finger/thumb squeezing movement.

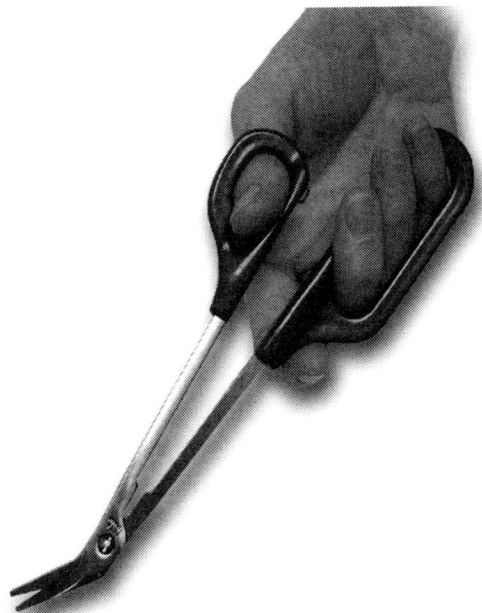

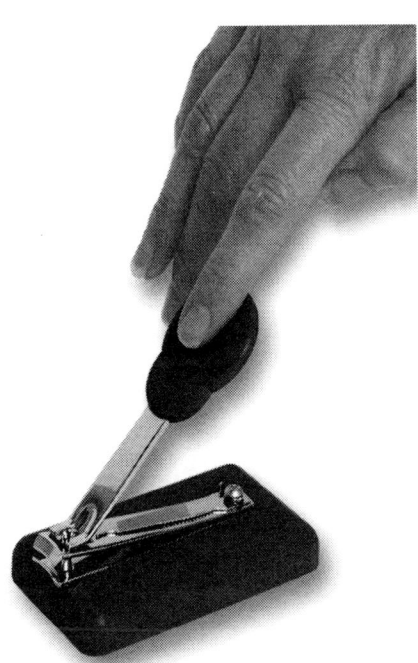

Figure 6.10 These nail clippers are mounted on a plastic base with non-slip feet. The finger pad gives good leverage and may be used with the downward pressure of three fingers on the pad.

Figure 6.9 Toe nail cutters which have an extended shank providing a long reach for people who have difficulty bending down to reach the toe nails. They have a long loop to accommodate three fingers, thus increasing control.

Where there is any danger of self injury because of tremor, dystonia, unsteadiness or lack of power of any kind, it is best to have someone to undertake manicures and pedicures. In such circumstances, it is best to dissuade the person from any attempt to cut their own nails whether it is with scissors, a nail clipper or even specially adapted tools.

Scissors for food preparation

Although many professional chefs would denounce the use of scissors instead of knives for food preparation, they are very useful for many people. Using scissors is the preferred method for some people for jointing chicken, snipping rather than chopping herbs and dicing bacon. Those who lack the power to wield a knife or who have visual problems may prefer to use scissors. Designated kitchen scissors are available in hardware and department stores. They usually have a notch near the screw end of the blades which allows small bones such as those in chicken to be severed. People who find these scissors difficult to use may like to keep a pair of their preferred scissors solely for kitchen use.

Cutting fabric

Cutting out a garment using a paper pattern, prior to sewing it, can be a daunting task. Sufficient time should be allowed for this process; in fact, some would say that planning the layout and cutting out of the pattern pieces can be a task equal to that of sewing the garment. Assuming that instructions such as using double or single fabric and following the grain or the bias of the fabric have been followed, there are several other points to consider more directly concerned with cutting the garment pieces. Straight pins, which are used to secure the paper pattern, should have their points directed towards the edge of the paper pattern piece. This allows the paper pattern to be smoothed absolutely flat on the fabric so that the pattern piece is accurately cut out. The surface on which the fabric is placed should be accessible from all sides; a table is more suitable than a worktop. The person who is cutting should stand with the non-scissor hand nearest to the table and that hand should be placed flat on top of the paper pattern and the fabric. The scissors should point in the direction in which the cut is to be made. Each cut should be as long and as smooth as possible. Where possible, each change of direction should begin from the edge of the pattern piece. Greater accuracy will be achieved in this way, avoiding negotiating corners and acute changes of direction with the scissor blades.

Scissors known as pinking shears are often used for finishing the edges of seams of non-fray fabrics as well as for decorative effects on craft materials such as felt. These scissors have blades which cut the fabric in a zigzag fashion. Pinking shears can also be used to produce this effect on paper or card, although it is best not to use the same pair for cutting both paper and fabric. There are also craft scissors whose blades produce various fancy edges (Figure 6.11).

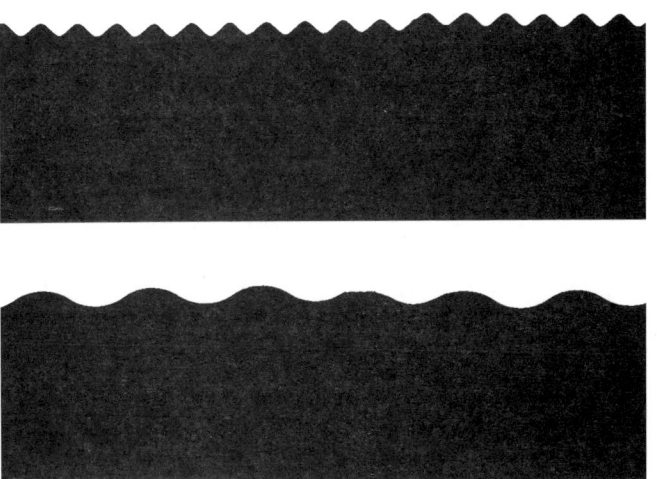

Figure 6.11 The zigzag edge produced with pinking sheers and two fancy edges produced by novelty blade craft scissors.

Maintenance of scissors

Scissors should be sharpened as often as is necessary. It is simple to have right-handed scissors sharpened, as sharpening machines are set to hone right-handed blades. There may be some difficulty having left-handed blades sharpened; they may need to be sent away for special treatment and take some time to be returned.

CHAPTER 7

Grading scissors activities

Correct scissors technique

As we have seen, the effective use of scissors usually requires two hands, one to handle the scissors and the other to control the material being cut. In the first instance, control of the scissors is paramount and the reciprocal action of opening and closing the blades must be undertaken without conscious effort; the movement must be automatic.

Some small children will prefer to use both hands to activate the scissors, using one hand for each scissors handle. Chapter 6 described the many types and sizes of scissors which are available, and the most appropriate ones must be chosen before the child can learn to manipulate them with one hand. Whether the child is using conventional scissors, self-opening ones with a spring or ones which require a whole-hand grip, the overall position of the hand is the same.

The hand should be in a position midway between pronation and supination, the thumb being uppermost. The wrist should be midway between flexion and extension. The forearm should be facing away from the body at right angles to it. One of the few exceptions to this position of the forearm and wrist is when cutting out a garment from a pattern laid on top of fabric. Another exception would be a person who has a deformity of the arm, wrist or hand.

If conventional scissors are being used, it is important to adopt an optimum grip with the hand in a position midway between pronation and supination as described above. It follows that the thumb will be uppermost whether the right hand or the left hand is used. The thumb is placed through the smaller of the two handles. The middle finger should be through the other handle and the index finger should be at the base of the handle so that it can help with closing the blades (Figure 7.1). Alternatively both the index and middle fingers may be placed through the handle. These finger positions are preferable to having the index finger only through the handle because the described positions afford more control

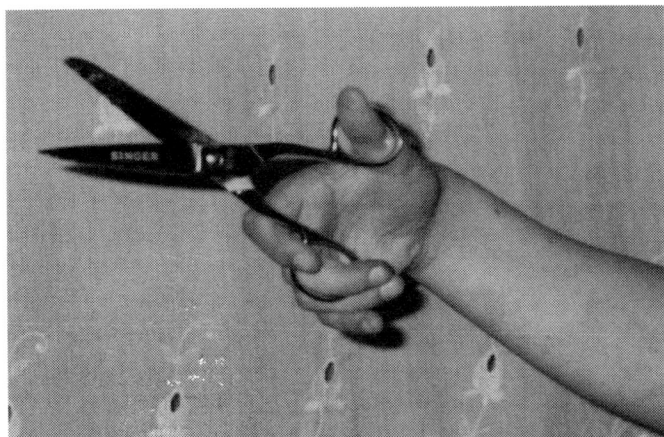

Figure 7.1 A good grip for conventional right-handed scissors. The thumb is through one loop and the middle finger is through the other loop with the index finger outside the loop helping to close the blades.

of the scissors. Large and heavy scissors will usually have a larger handle to accommodate all the fingers.

Whichever type of scissors is being used, the blades should point away from the body. Usually it is the material in the non-scissors hand which moves to allow accurate cutting.

Special consideration should be given to people who suffer from hemiplegia. Firstly they may hold the scissors in what was their non-preferred hand and thus have some difficulty with this and many other fine hand skills. This is an important consideration whether the hemiplegia is congenital or acquired. With children it may be difficult to decide which hand would have been dominant had the child not suffered from hemiplegia. The possibility that what would have been the non-preferred or non-dominant hand may be used as the preferred one should be borne in mind, and the possibility of the hand used being not quite as agile as would be expected should be considered. In adult-acquired hemiplegia it will be clear whether the preferred or non-preferred hand is being used.

The second consideration is that the material being cut will, perforce, be held in the hemiplegic hand, which has increased tone and may have poor tactile sensation. Often there is difficulty controlling the hand unless it is visually monitored. This need to look at the hemiplegic hand leaves little vision free to monitor the cutting process. Because of increased tone, the hand may begin by holding the paper, or other material, satisfactorily, but as the activity proceeds an increase in muscle tone may occur which causes the material to be spoiled. This problem can, in some instances, be removed by holding materials such as paper in a large sprung clothes peg or similar gripper. In this way the paper is not spoiled and the sprung peg is held with a whole hand grip, rather than a fingers and thumb grip (Figure 7.2).

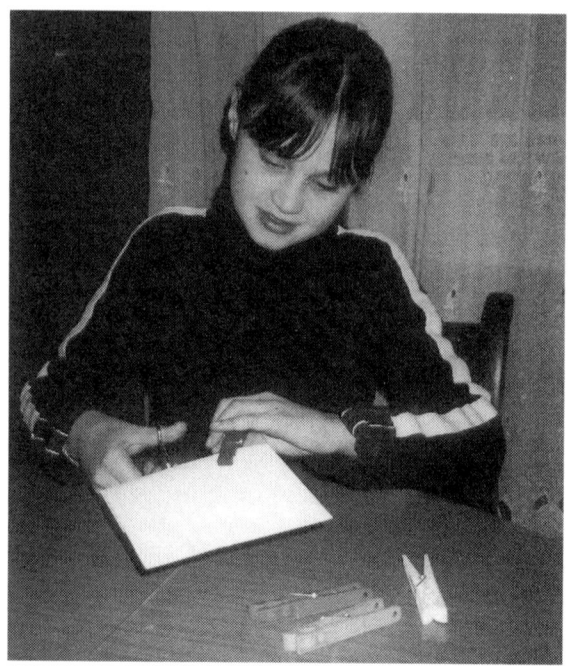

Figure 7.2 Where there is increased tone in the hand holding the paper it is sometimes better to grip the paper in a spring clothes peg and hold the peg rather than the paper. This prevents the paper being crumpled.

Some children and adults who have virtually only one hand to use effectively for scissors activities have been observed cutting paper quite effectively with the paper supported on a table or other flat surface. The little finger side of their scissors hand is used to steady the paper. Sometimes it is possible to steady the paper with the non-scissors hand (Figure 7.3).

To be most effective, the blades of the scissors should be at right angles to the material which is being cut (Figure 7.4). If this is not so, the blades will not cut the material easily. Children sometimes complain that scissors will not cut, when all that is needed is for the relative positions of the scissors blades and the material being cut to be adjusted so that the blades and the material are at right angles to each other. Of course, there are instances when children are trying to cut with scissors that are genuinely blunt!

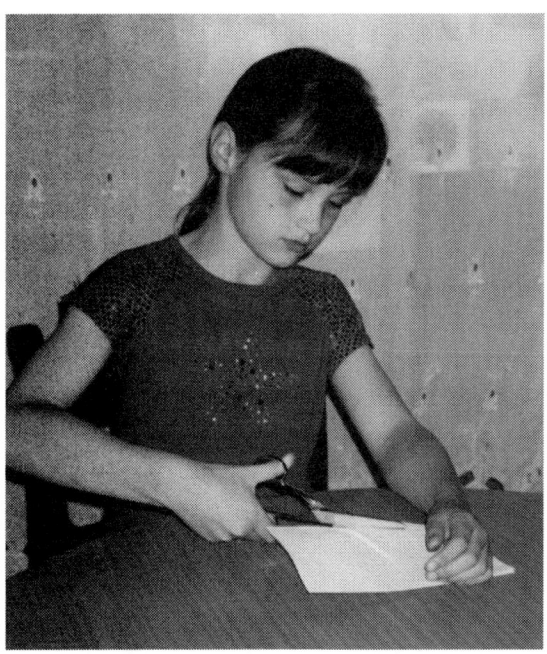

Figure 7.3 Here the paper is resting on the work surface and the non-scissors hand is steadying the paper.

Figure 7.4 Joanna is holding the card she will cut parallel to the table and the blades of the scissors are positioned at right angles to the card.

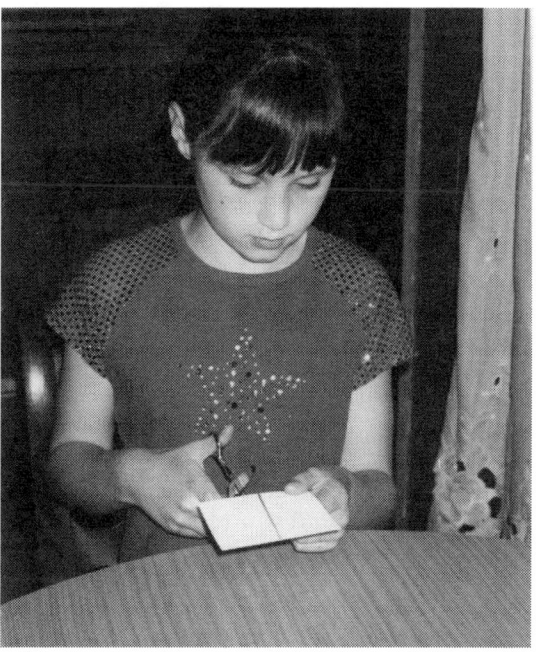

A selection of graded scissors activities

After learning to hold the scissors in the correct manner, learning to snip, with the type of scissors most appropriate for the user, is the next step. The material used will depend on the developmental age and skill. Sometimes, in the early stages of working with young children, cylinders of Playdoh® or Plasticene® or other modelling clay may be used (Figure 7.5). Playdoh® provides the least resistance to the scissors blades. Various types of modelling clay will provide different degrees of resistance and should be chosen according to the muscle power of the child. A greater degree of resistance may help those with some unsteadiness of the hand.

Figure 7.5 Alice is enjoying snipping modelling clay to practise reciprocal scissors movements before using strips of card for her first real cutting activity.

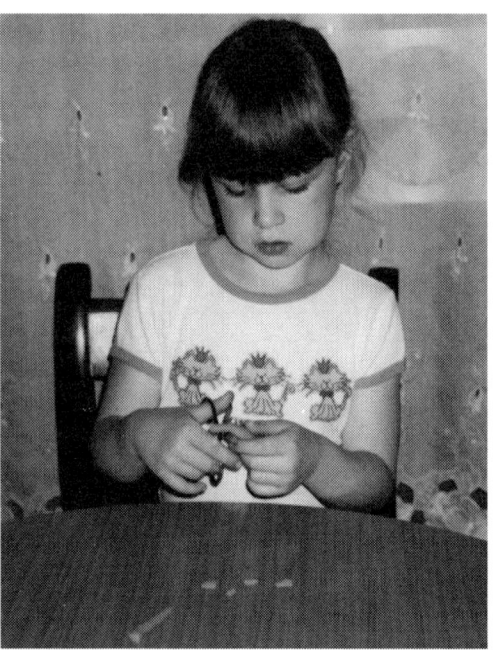

Generally thin card is easier to cut than paper; the former has more rigidity and is less likely to bend round the blades of the scissors. For first attempts at cutting, narrow strips of card, perhaps between 3 and 5 cm wide, are ideal because the strip can be cut completely with one snip of the scissors. Many printers will be glad to give away their off-cuts of card, which are often attractively coloured.

Initially just snipping bits of the card will be pleasing to most children. The author has treated many children who have carefully gathered up the cut bits of card and taken every one of them home to be treasured. At this stage the snipping of card or paper is the process which brings satisfaction to the young child. This is similar to the way that first attempts at painting with a brush will be simply applying paint to paper; no attempt will be made to produce a picture of any kind. This is an important stage in learning to cut with scissors, where the actual process of manipulating the scissors is learned.

The next step is learning to cut in a specific position on the strips of card. Begin with drawing a wide 'road' or 'path' across the card. The 'road' should be sufficiently wide and boldly drawn to ensure success. Gradually the 'roads' can be narrower, as cutting becomes more accurate, until the child is able to cut along a heavy line. To allow for more cuts across the card, increase the width of the card or draw cutting lines diagonally across it. Depending on the direction of the diagonal lines, triangles or rhombi will be cut (see Worksheets 1 and 2).

An activity of interest to many children is making a 'crown' from card. This is a further activity involving cutting short diagonal lines whilst at the same time learning to stop each cut at a specific point. Each cut is started at the edge of the card (see Worksheet 3).

When the process of cutting along a short straight line has been mastered, cutting out straight-sided shapes can be attempted. The most appropriate shapes for first attempts are various types of triangles, gradually increasing in size so that increasingly longer lines are cut. Each side of the triangle should be started from the edge of the paper or card so that the blades of the scissors never have to change direction. This is an important point for all scissors activities: where possible, cuts are begun from the edge of the material, thus removing the need for the scissors blades to change direction, especially where the change of direction is an acute angle.

Further practice could be gained with cutting out other straight-sided shapes such as squares and rectangles, which can be used to build houses, windows, doors and other buildings, as well as flags, which can be coloured after cutting out (see Worksheets 4 and 5).

Seasonal straight-sided shapes such as stars, candles and triangular Christmas trees can be made with paper and later coloured with paint, felt-tipped pens or crayons. Alternatively coloured paper or card may be used.

A tip for older children and adults when cutting a straight line, is to set the scissors pointing towards the end of the line and keep the eye focused on the end of the line. For most people this results in an acceptably straight cut. Where the line which is to be cut is reasonably long, cuts involving almost the whole length of the scissors blade produce a clean cut. Using many small cuts will result in an uneven cut.

The converse is true when cutting a curved line; in this case, the cuts should be controlled and short. The material being cut is constantly moved to facilitate following the curve with the blades of the scissors. This is a skilled manoeuvre which requires concentration, visual attention to the line being cut and unconscious, automatic movements to control the scissors and move the material being cut appropriately.

Cutting activities should always be purposeful. Where possible there should always be an end product, however simple.

Graded projects

1. A very simple disposable glue spreader can be made by snipping along a length of paper. It is then rolled up and secured with adhesive tape (see Worksheet 6).

2. Using coloured or patterned paper, or even paper which the child has crayoned or painted, a very simple lantern can be made. Depending on the skill of the child these may be very small, to hang on a Christmas tree, or larger, to use as a single decoration. A piece of paper is folded in two lengthways and cuts are made from the folded edge to almost the opposite edge. A bold line will indicate how deeply the cuts should be made. According to skill of the child, the cuts may be made freely or along lines provided. The 'lantern' is then joined along the shorter sides with glue, adhesive tape or staples. A paper handle is then added (see Worksheet 7).

3. A woven mat provides scissors practice similar to the lantern activity and also practice in cutting strips of paper. A square of paper is folded in two and equidistant cuts made from the folded edge almost to the opposite edge. Strips of paper are cut the same length as one side of square and the same width as the distance between the cuts on the square of paper. The strips are then 'woven' between the cuts on the square of paper. This activity may be

very simple, with only three or five cuts and two or four strips, or as complex as the child's skill and imagination allows. Fairly strong paper which does not tear very easily will be best. Other materials could be used for the weaving, such as flattened drinking straws, scraps of tape and braid, thick string or knitting yarn. The ends of the weaving are secured with glue, double-sided adhesive tape or Sticky Fixers®.

4. A simple but very effective three-dimensional Christmas tree can made from two triangles of card. Small versions may be hung on a Christmas tree or a number may made into a mobile. Larger versions may be decorated and used as table decorations (see Worksheet 8).

5. Cutting geometric shapes and making pictures (see Worksheet 9).

6. Practising cutting curves is more interesting if there is a finished product. Worksheet 10 describes how to make a spiral mobile.

7. A house with an opening door and windows requires accurate cutting and, later, folding to open the door and windows (see Worksheet 11).

8. Most people are interested in making strings of motifs by folding paper concertina-wise and cutting through all the layers of paper at once. Care must be taken to ensure that the motifs remain attached to each other at some point, either at each side or at the top and bottom. Worksheets 12 and 13 provide two examples of such projects.

9. Flower shapes may cut from circles of paper (see Worksheet 14). Several layers of tissue paper may be used to create three-dimensional flowers. More complex shapes may be used with more and differently shaped petals than the one in the given example. Flowers may have stems made from drinking straws or similar material. Small flowers may be used on the front of greetings cards. A posy of flowers would make a pleasing Mothers' Day present.

10. Most children enjoy making paper 'snowflakes'. These can be very simple or complex according to the child's skill (see Worksheet 15). They may be fashioned from a piece of paper folded into four, from which the corners are cut. More complex shapes may be cut allowing practice with cutting curves and corners. Do not fold the paper too many times or it will be difficult to cut. If more cut outs are needed to make a pattern the paper may be refolded to expose different edges. This activity can be adjusted for various seasons of the year by making the results into doilies to place under cakes on a plate. Several small ones may be stapled together to make a 'flower' which may be mounted on a drinking straw 'stem' or several may be used to make a picture.

11. Masks can be made from a shaped piece of paper or card with holes cut for the eyes, nose and mouth. They may be made from coloured paper or card or painted, crayoned or decorated with stickers, fabric or woollen yarn. More ambitious masks may be made using paper sculpture and curled paper.

12. Handmade greetings cards are popular; they are commercially available although an increasing number of people enjoy making their own cards for family and friends. Simple designs are often the most effective. Materials for cards may be bought specially for the purpose, although scrap materials such as wrapping paper, bows, ribbons and metallic card from boxes and packaging can all be utilized for cards. See Worksheets 16–18 for three simple but effective designs.

When the use of scissors is not a realistic aim

For some people, scissors skills will never be a realistic possibility. Some children will never possess the necessary muscle power, whilst others will never have sufficient control of muscle tone. The latter could be as a result of cerebral palsy, ataxia or dystonia. Where these problems are severe it would be unkind to embark on a programme of learning scissors skills. For other children whose problems are not so severe, it may be difficult to decide if scissors skills will develop into a useful skill.

Some adults may never have used scissors; others may have acquired disabilities which make use of conventional scissors unrealistic and/or dangerous to the user or to other people. Using scissors may be contraindicated when there is joint inflammation or damage in conditions such as rheumatoid arthritis.

It is important to be realistic when assessing the appropriateness of teaching or relearning scissors skills. For some craft activities it may be more appropriate to choose paper tearing activities, perhaps using interesting handmade papers, rather than the person being disappointed with their poor scissors skills. Another possibility is the use of a paper trimmer to produce straight-sided shapes. There are small punches available which require only whole-hand pressure to cut out small shapes such as snowflakes, hearts, Christmas trees and stars. Designs can be made either with the shapes which are cut out or the silhouettes remaining in the paper from which the shapes are cut.

References

Armada Art (1998) www.armadart.com/scissatory.hmt

Barsley M (1966) The Left-Handed Book. An investigation into the sinister history of left-handedness. London: Souvenir Press Ltd.

Beery KE, Buktenica NA (1997) Developmental Test of Visual-Motor Integration (VMI). Cleveland: Modern Curriculum Press.

Bishop DVM (1990) Handedness and developmental disorder. Clinics in Developmental Medicine 110: 92–100.

Craft AW (1985) Arthritis in children. Paediatric Symposium. British Journal of Hospital Medicine 33(4):188–94.

Fahn S (1972) Differential diagnosis of tremors: symposium on clinical neurology. Medical Clinics of North America 6(6): 1363–75.

Gardner MF (1992) Test of Visual Perceptual Skills (non-motor) Upper Level. Seattle: Special Child Publications. Available in UK from Ann Arbor Publishers, PO Box 1, Belford, Northumberland, NE70 7JX.

Gardner MF (1996) Test of Visual Perceptual Skills (non-motor) Lower Level. Seattle: Special Child Publications. Available in UK from Ann Arbor Publishers, PO Box 1, Belford, Northumberland, NE70 7JX.

Hosking G (1982) An Introduction to Paediatric Neurology. London: Faber and Faber.

Jones K (1988) Smith's Recognisable Patterns of Human Malformation. Philadelphia, London, Toronto: WB Saunders.

Millidot (1986) Dictionary of Optometry. London: Butterworth.

Opie I, Opie P (1992) The Oxford Dictionary of Nursery Rhymes. Oxford: Oxford University Press.

Opie I, Opie P (1997) Children's Games and Things. Oxford: Oxford University Press.

Paul D (1997) Living Left-handed. London: Bloomsbury Publishing plc.

Penso DE (1987) Occupational Therapy for Children with Disabilities. London: Croom Helm; Rockville, Maryland: Aspen Publishers, Inc.

Penso DE (1992) The mucopolysaccharidoses:classification, symptoms and the role of the occupational therapist. British Journal of Occupational Therapy 55(2): 44–8.

Penso DE (1993) Perceptuo-Motor Difficulties: theory and strategies to help children, adolescents and adults. London: Chapman and Hall; distributed in USA and Canada by Singular Publishing Company, Inc., San Diego, California.

Penso DE (1999) Keyboarding Skills for Children with Disabilities. London: Whurr Publishers.

Turner A (1996) The Practice of Occupational Therapy: an introduction to the treatment of physical dysfunction. London: Churchill Livingstone.

Williams HG (1983) Perceptual and Motor Development. New Jersey: Prentice-Hall.

Further reading

Ansell B (1981) When Your Child has Arthritis. London: Arthritis and Rheumatism Council for Research.

Beran R (1982) Learning about Epilepsy. Oxford: Medical Information Services Limited.

Brown B, Henderson S (1989) A sloping desk? Should the wheel turn full circle? Handwriting Review 3: 55-9.

Colley M (2000) Living with Dyspraxia: a guide for adults with developmental dyspraxia. Hitchin: The Dyspraxia Foundation Adult Support Group.

Diagnosing and Teaching Scissors Skills (1976) Developmental Learning Materials.

Finnie N (1997) Handling the Young Cerebral Palsied Child at Home. Oxford: Butterworth Heinemann.

Handley J (1986) Posture education in primary schools. Health at School 1(6):176-7; 1(7): 220-1; 1(8): 259-60.

Haskell H, Barrett K (1989) The Education of Children with Motor and Neurological Disabilities. London: Chapman and Hall; New York: Nichols Publishing.

Hawkins S, Gadsby M (1991) Perceptuo-motor deficit: a major learning difficulty. British Journal of Occupational Therapy 54(4): 145-9.

Hoare D, Larking D (1991) Kinaesthetic abilities of clumsy children. Developmental and Child Neurology 33(6): 671-8.

Kashani J (1986) Self-esteem of handicapped children and adolescents. Developmental Medicine and Child Neurology 28(1): 77-83.

King-Thomas L, Hacker B (Eds) (1987) A Therapist's Guide to Paediatric Assessment. New York: Little Brown and Company.

Lee M, French J (undated) Dyspraxia – a handbook for therapists. London: Association of Paediatric Chartered Physiotherapists.

Losse H, Henderson S et al. (1991) Clumsiness in children – do they grow out of it? Developmental Medicine and Child Neurology 33(1): 55-68.

McKinlay I (1987) Children with motor learning difficulties: not so much a syndrome - more a way of life. Physiotherapy 73(11): 653-8.

Mahoney S, Markwell A (1997) Developing Scissor Skills - A guide for parents and teachers. Dunmow: Peta (UK) Ltd.

Marsh N (1998) Start to Finish: developmentally sequenced fine motor activities for preschool children. Bisbee, Arizona: Imaginart International, Inc.

Myers P (1987) The sloping board. Handwriting Review 1: 43.

Poustie J (1997) Solutions for Specific Learning Difficulties. Taunton: Next Generation.

Restricted Growth Association (1989) The Layman's Guide to Restricted Growth. Hayling Island, Hampshire: Restricted Growth Association.

Tyerman A (undated) Psychological Effects of Head Injury. Nottingham: Headway, The National Head Injuries Association.

Glossary

Accommodation, visual The process by which the eye focuses on an object. This is brought about by the movement of the eye muscles which adjust the curvature and thickness of the lens.

Amblyopia A condition characterized by low visual acuity without any apparent lesion of the eye or proven disorder of the visual pathways and which is not correctable by optical means.

Apposition Placing next to, as in finger/thumb apposition, placing the thumb and finger next to each other to produce a finger/thumb grip.

Apraxia The inability to plan movements mentally prior to their execution.

Associated movements Unintended movements which accompany intended movements. For example, a child's early attempts at writing with a pencil may be accompanied by tongue movements which roughly mirror the movements of the hand.

Ataxia Lack of muscle coordination which causes jerky, unsteady movements.

Athetosis Involuntary writhing movements due to cerebral malfunction. A symptom of one type of cerebral palsy.

Atlanto-axial joint The joint between the first two vertebrae (bones) of the spinal column (the backbone). The first vertebra, the atlas, supports the globe of the head. The second vertebra, the axis, provides the pivot upon which the atlas and, with it, the skull rotates.

Binocular vision When both eyes contribute towards producing a percept.

Cerebellum (*Adjective* cerebellar) The part of the brain at the back of the head which lies beneath the cerebrum (the large part of the brain occupying most of the skull) and above the medulla oblongata (the part of the spinal cord which lies within the skull). The cerebellum coordinates impulses from the organs of balance and from the joints. It monitors impulses coming from the brain to ensure that the movement follows the intended path. It maintains the normal tone of the muscles by its action on the brainstem. Damage to the cerebellum results in an unsteady gait, incoordination and hypotonia (low muscle tone).

Cerebral cortex The external layer of the cerebrum, the largest area of the brain, which is divided into the right and left hemispheres.

Cerebrovascular accident (CVA) Temporary or permanent damage to part of the brain caused by haemorrhage, a blood clot in a cerebral blood vessel, or physical damage to part of the brain. The effects of the damage will depend on the area of the brain which is involved, the effect being manifested on the opposite side of the body to the site of the damage. Vision and language may also be involved. Other names for CVA include stroke and seizure.

Congenital Present at birth.

Connective tissue Tissue which supports and connects organs and structures of the body. The term is often used to describe the tissue round joints.

Contracture Permanent contraction of a part of the body, most usually occurring in the upper or lower limb, which is caused by the formation of inelastic fibrous tissue.

Cranial Of the skull or cranium.

Distal Situated furthest from the centre of the body. For example, the final joints of the fingers are the distal joints.

Dycem® A non-slip material which is available either on a roll, which can then be cut to the required size and shape, or in the form of ready-made mats of various sizes. Dycem® may be used to prevent all manner of objects from slipping including paper, books, computers, dishes and plates.

Dyspraxia Difficulty with planning and organizing movements at a cerebral level. Dyspraxia can affect any or all executive skills from self-help activities to handwriting and speech.

Dystonia Abnormal, fluctuating muscle tone.

Epilepsy An epileptic attack is due to a transitory disturbance of the function of the brain. It is a paroxysmal and transitory disturbance due to excessive neuronal discharge in the brain. There are a number of types of seizure, including tonic-clonic attacks (grand mal), petit mal, temporal lobe attacks, focal epilepsy and myoclonic epilepsy (Hosking 1982).

Epiphysis (plural epiphyses) The end of a long bone developed separately but attached by cartilage to the shaft of the bone. It is at this junction between the epiphysis and the shaft that growth takes place. When growth is complete the epiphysis unites with the shaft of the bone.

Flexion Bending of any part of the body.

Hand–eye coordination The appreciation that the object held or manipulated by the hand is the same one which is observed by the eyes, thus hand and eye are able to work together on a particular activity.

Hemiplegia Paralysis or partial paralysis of one side of the body.

In utero In the uterus. The term usually refers to a child before birth.

Kyphosis The term refers to an abnormal curve of the spinal column in a posterior direction giving a humpbacked appearance. Sometimes the curvature is in both a posterior and a lateral direction when it is known as a kyphoscoliosis.

Lordosis An abnormal forward curve of the spine in the lumbar region (lower back), giving a hollow-backed appearance.

Lumbar Pertaining to the loins.

Metacarpophalangeal joint The joint between the hand and the fingers defined by the knuckles.

Motor effect Movement, voluntary or involuntary, conscious or unconscious, that takes place as the consequence of sensory input which has been perceived and understood.

Motor learning difficulties Problems with learning the skills of movement in the absence of general sensory and intellectual handicaps. A further criterion is that there are no hard neurological signs. Other terms which have been used for this condition are clumsy child syndrome, developmental coordination disorder and (erroneously) dyspraxia.

Myelin The fatty covering of some nerves.

Nystagmus A regular, repetitive and involuntary movement of the eye with variable direction, amplitude and frequency. The direction of these abnormal eye movements may be vertical, horizontal, diagonal or rotatory. People with a nystagmus will usually find the fields of vision where the nystagmus is least troublesome and hold their head in such a position that these optimum fields of vision are used.

Occupational therapist A professionally qualified person who treats physical and psychiatric conditions through specific activities in order to help people reach their maximum level of function and independence in all aspects of daily life.

Orthoses Splints used to support, prevent strain, maintain position and correct deformity of body parts.

Orthotist A person skilled in the manufacture of orthoses or splints.

Paramedical Beside or ancillary to the medical. Therapists are sometimes described as paramedical.

Paraplegia Paralysis of the lower limbs and lower part of the trunk.

Perinatal Around the time of birth which includes the period before birth, birth and the period following birth.

Peripheral vision Vision resulting from stimulation of the retina outside the fovea, a condition in which only the outer parts of the retina are stimulated.

Physiotherapist A person who treats disease, disability or injury by physical means, most usually by active methods requiring the cooperation of the person being treated. It is concerned with the maintenance of posture and active movement.

Plantigrade The position of the foot in which the whole of the sole is in contact with the floor or other horizontal surface.

Pronation Turning the palm of the hand downwards.

Proprioception Awareness of posture, balance and position. This is due to receptors (called proprioceptors) located within muscles, tendons, joints and the vestibular system apparatus of the inner ear (Millidot 1986).

Reciprocal movements Back and forth movements such as those used when brushing the teeth, polishing shoes or using a grater.

Refractive disorders (of the eye) These are conditions in which there is relaxed accommodation and the image of objects at infinity is not formed on the retina. The result is blurred vision. Conditions in which this type of visual error occurs are astigmatism, hypermetropia and myopia.

Retinitis pigmentosa An inherited disease of the eye which is characterized by night blindness and constricted visual fields. The condition usually affects both eyes.

Sclerosis Hardening caused by the overgrowth of fibrous or connective tissue.

Scoliosis An abnormal curvature of the spine in a lateral direction. Sometimes the curvature is in both a posterior and a lateral direction when it is known as a kyphoscoliosis. See also **lordosis**.

Spasm (muscle) A sudden involuntary contraction of one or more muscles. Muscle spasm is a symptom of cerebral palsy which greatly affects coordinated movements.

Spina bifida Incomplete fusion of part of the spinal column which leaves the spinal cord exposed or partially exposed.

Supination Turning the palm of the hand upwards.

Symptom A term applied to any evidence of a disease; strictly it is applied to subjective evidence of the person who is experiencing the symptoms. The term 'sign' is usually applied to symptoms of which the patient does not complain but which are elicited upon physical examination.

Syndrome A group of symptoms or characteristics, all or most of which occur in a particular disorder.

Thoracic Relating to the thorax.

Tone The normal degree of tension in a muscle.

Trauma A wound or injury.

Tremor An involuntary trembling of voluntary muscles (those used for movement). The amplitude of the tremor may vary from very fine (10–12 vibrations per second) to coarse. The characteristics of tremors are various and include intention tremor where the tremor intensifies when movement is attempted.

Vestibular apparatus The part of the inner ear concerned with balance.

Visual acuity The capacity for seeing distinctly the details of an object.

Visual fields The extent of space in which objects are visible to an eye in a given position. The visual field extends to approximately 100 degrees horizontally outwards, 60 degrees nasally, 65 degrees upwards and 75 degrees downwards when the eye is in a straight forward position.

Useful addresses

College of Occupational Therapists Ltd
106–114 Borough High Street
Southwark
London SE1 1LB
Tel: 020 7357 6480

Dyspraxia Foundation
8 West Alley
Hitchin
Hertfordshire SG5 1EG
Tel: 01462 455016

National Association of Paediatric Occupational Therapists (NAPOT)
Professional Briefings
37a Star Street
Ware
Hertfordshire SG12 7AA
Tel: 01920 469 083

Nottingham Rehab Ltd.
Findel House
Excelsior Road
Ashby Park
Ashby de la Zouch
Leicestershire LE 65 1NG
Tel: 0845 606 0911

Distributors in USA
Access-Ability
610 Sample Road
Pompano Beach
Florida FL 33064
USA
Tel: 954 942 1882

Peta (UK) Ltd
Mark's Hall
Mark's Hall Lane
Margaret Roding
Dunmow CM6 1QT
Tel: 01245 231 118

Distributors in USA
Mecanaids Co Inc
21 Hampden Drive
South Easton
MA 02375
USA
Tel: 1 800 227 0877

The Left-Handed Company
Dept LH
PO Box52
South DO
Manchester M 20 2P
Tel: 0161 445 0159

Fred Sammons Inc
Box 32
Brookfield
Illinois 60513
USA
Tel: 1 800 323 5547

Worksheets

Worksheet 1

Template for card strips with graded widths of 'roads' along which to cut.

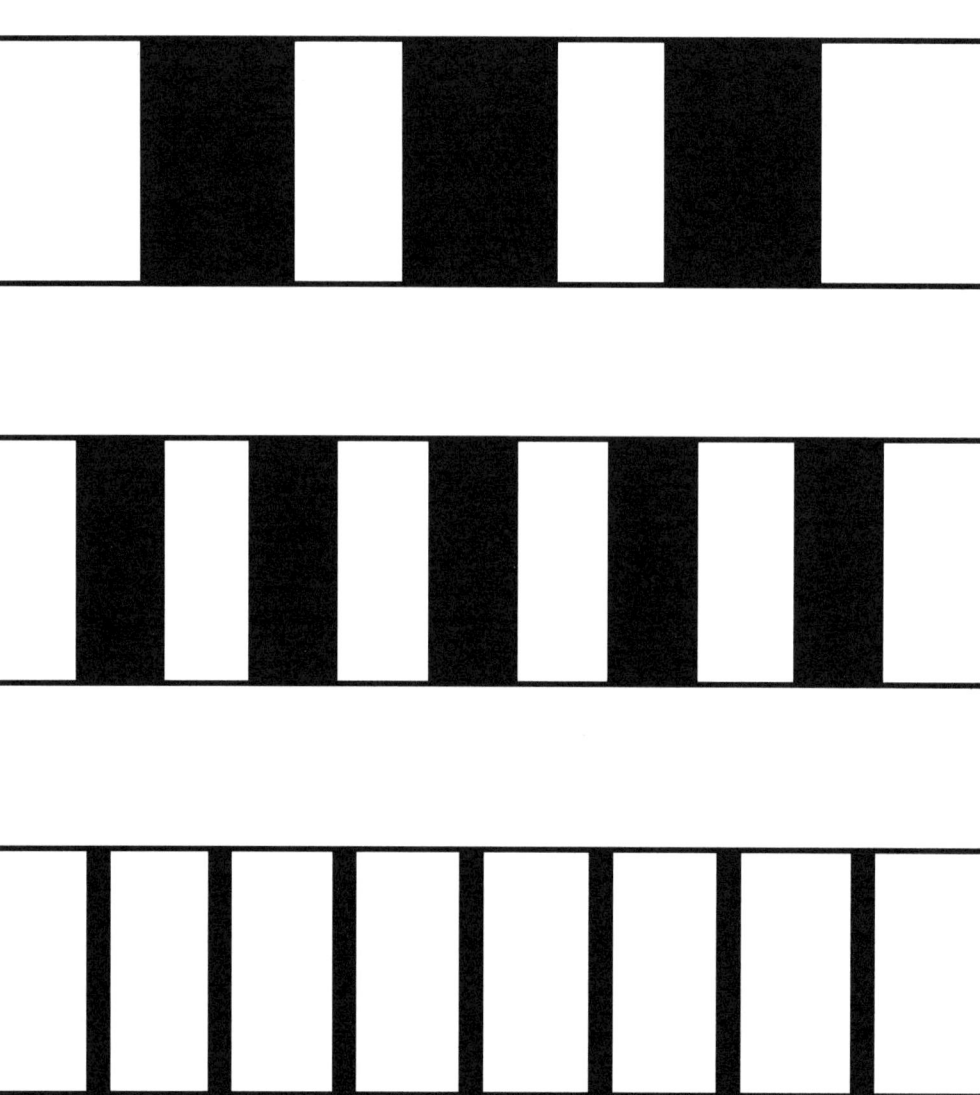

Worksheet 2

Template for card strips with diagonal lines which will form triangles and rhombi. If strips of various colours are used these shapes may be used to make mosaic patterns.

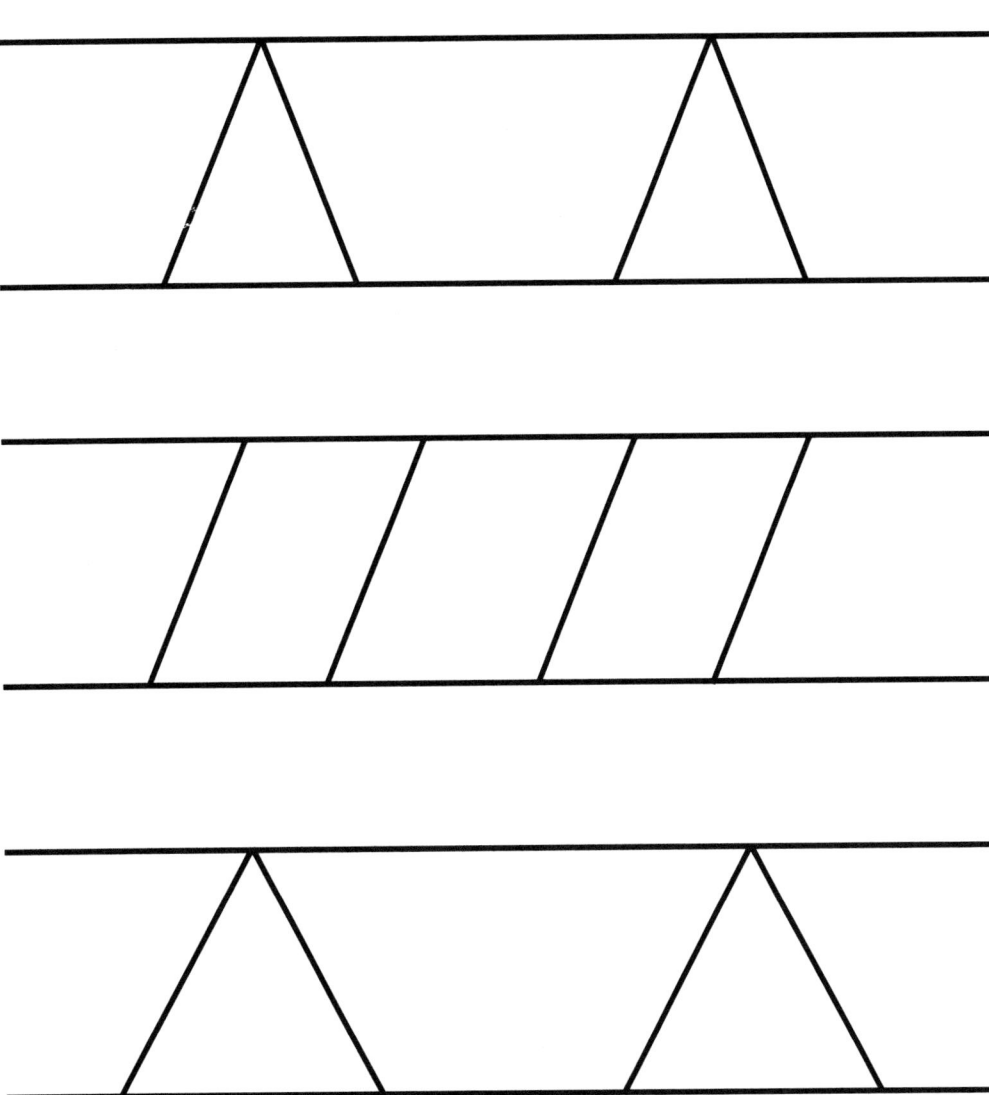

Worksheet 3

Template for making a card crown. The pattern should be continued until long enough to encircle the head and provide an overlap for joining into a circle. Make it simply from coloured card or it may be elaborately painted and 'jewelled'. Start each cut from the points of the crown. Do not attempt to turn any corners with the scissors.

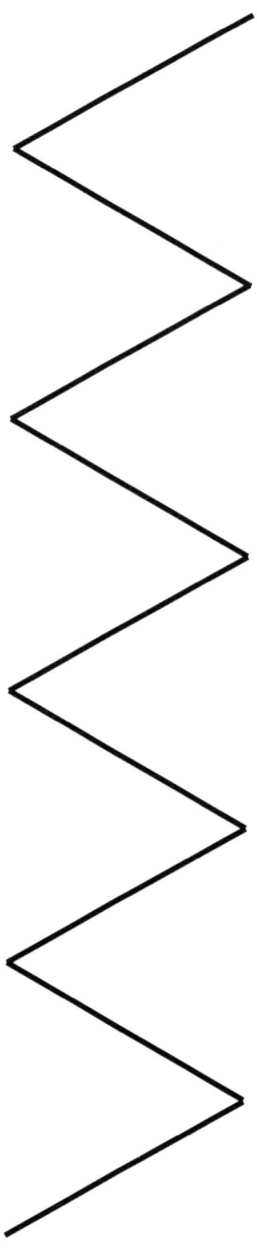

Worksheet 4

Straight-sided shapes which may be combined to make a variety of pictures such as houses, bridges, shops etc. For people who are developing scissors skills each shape should be separated from the others before it is cut out.

Worksheet 5

More straight-sided shapes to combine to make buildings, robots etc. For people who are developing scissors skills each shape should be separated from the others before it is cut out.

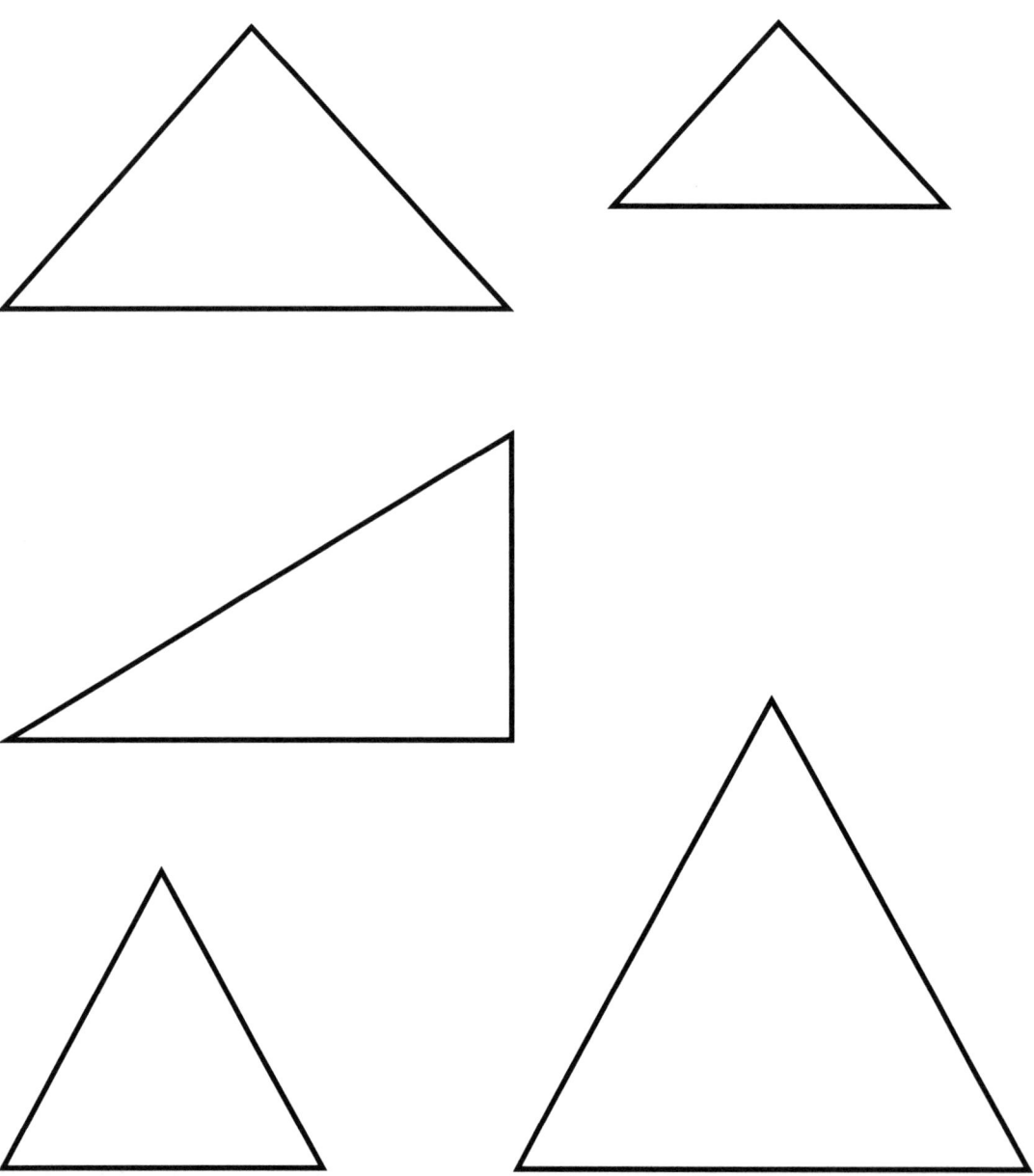

Worksheet 6

A simple glue spreader made from a fringed strip of paper. Cut along the dotted lines then roll up and secure the handle with adhesive tape. The cuts need not be accurate; therefore it makes a good first project to attempt where success is assured.

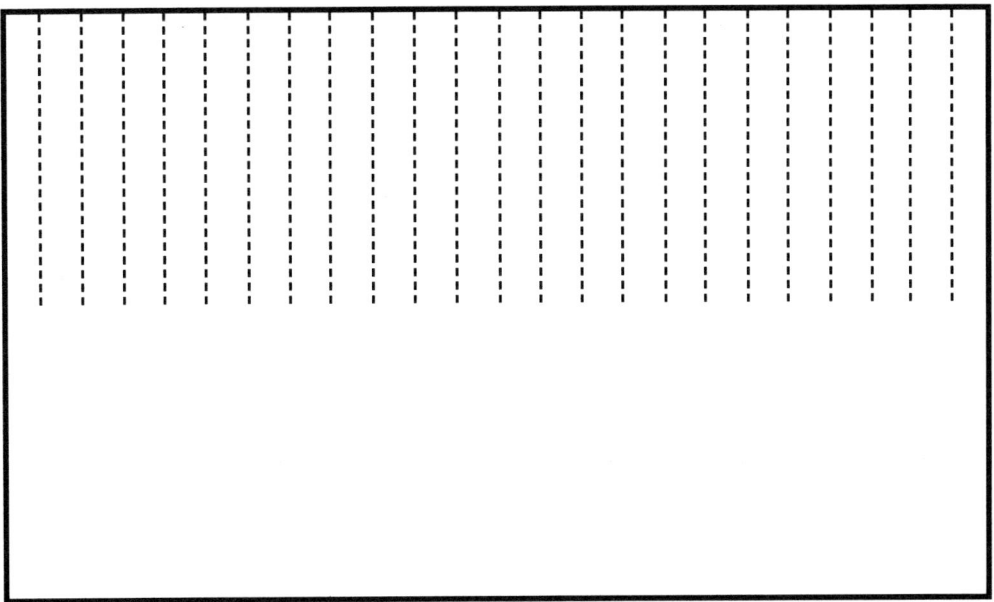

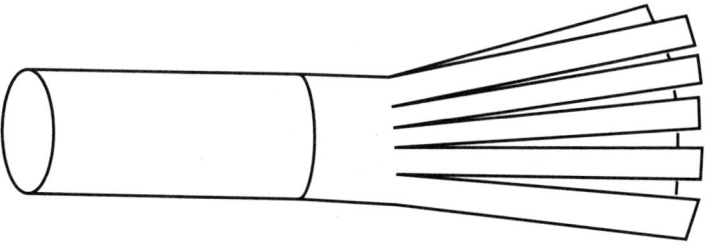

Worksheet 7

A simple paper lantern made from a folded piece of paper with cuts made along the dotted lines. It could be made from coloured paper or decorated with felt tip pens and glitter. Small lanterns may be hung on a Christmas tree or a number could be arranged to make a mobile.

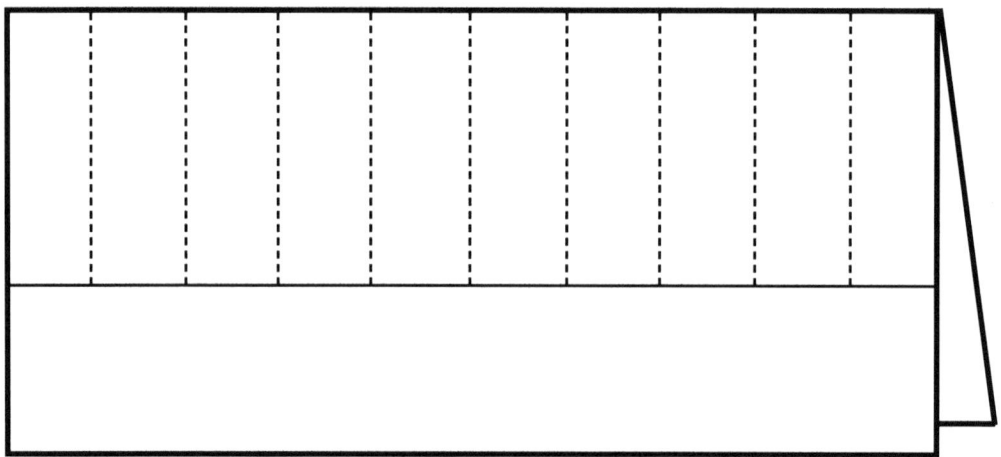

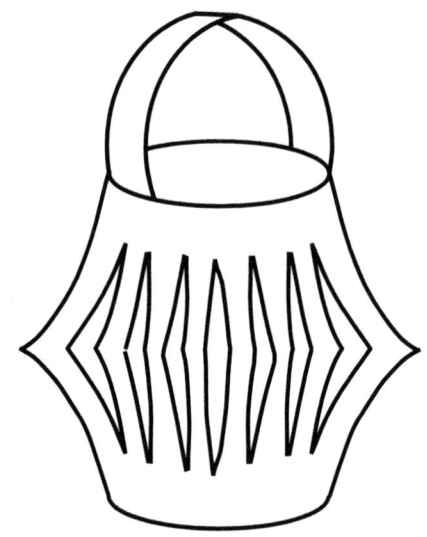

Worksheet 8

Template used to make a three-dimensional card Christmas tree. Two triangles are cut out and slots cut along the illustrated dotted lines. The two parts are then slotted together.

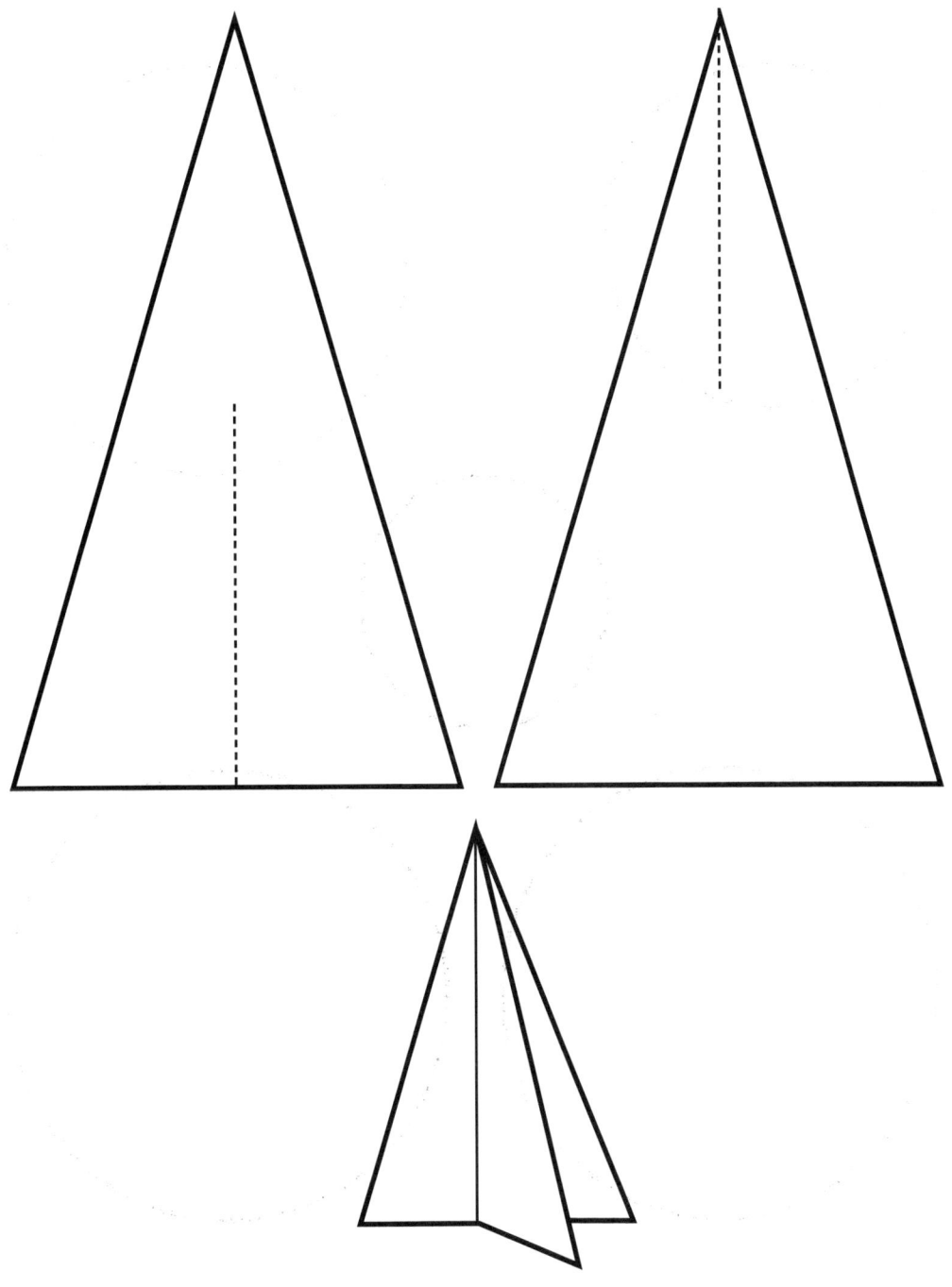

Worksheet 9

Templates of circles which can be used to make wheels, faces or as the basis for flowers or snowflake patterns. Note that the smaller the circle the more difficult it will be to cut out accurately.

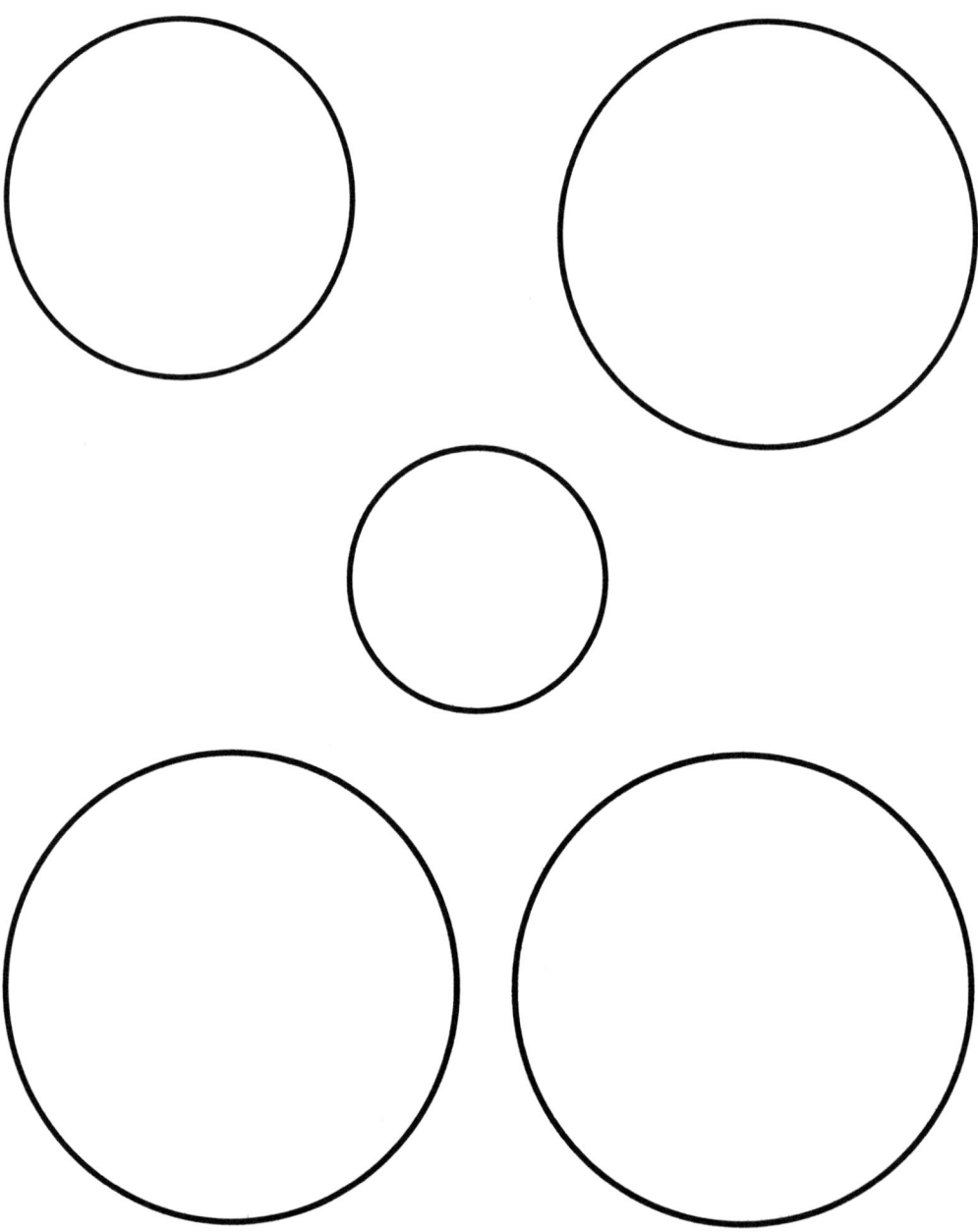

Worksheet 10

Cutting spirals provides practice with curves. If the spiral is cut from metallic refractory card it makes an attractive mobile. It should be threaded with strong thread or fine string through the centre and the outer spiral so it may be hung to gyrate in a draught of air. The same shape may also be coloured to represent a snake.

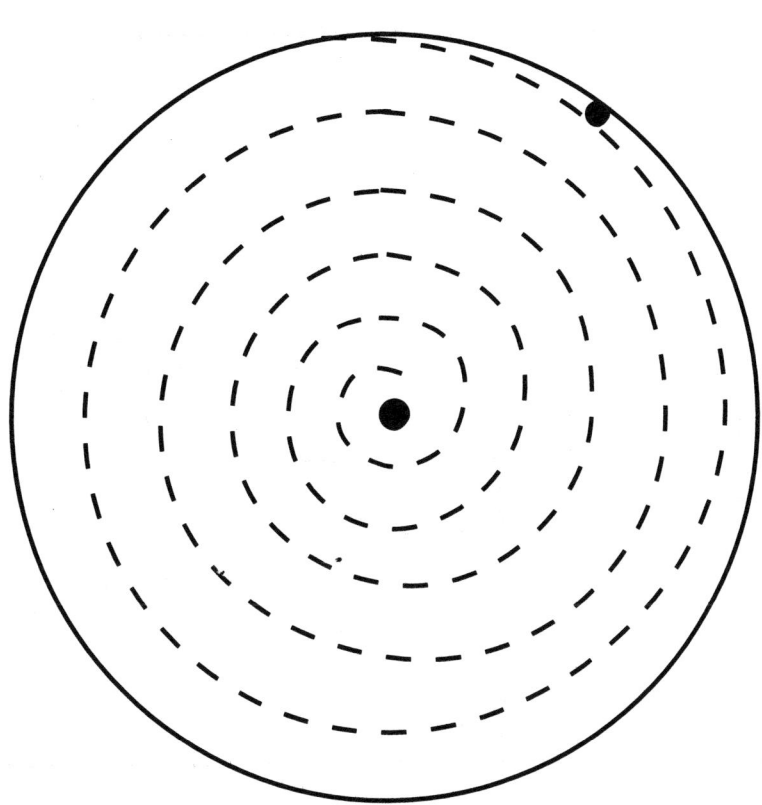

Worksheet 11

A house with a door and windows which can be opened. Cut on the dotted lines then fold the door and windows open. This activity provides good practice with scissors control and accurate cutting.

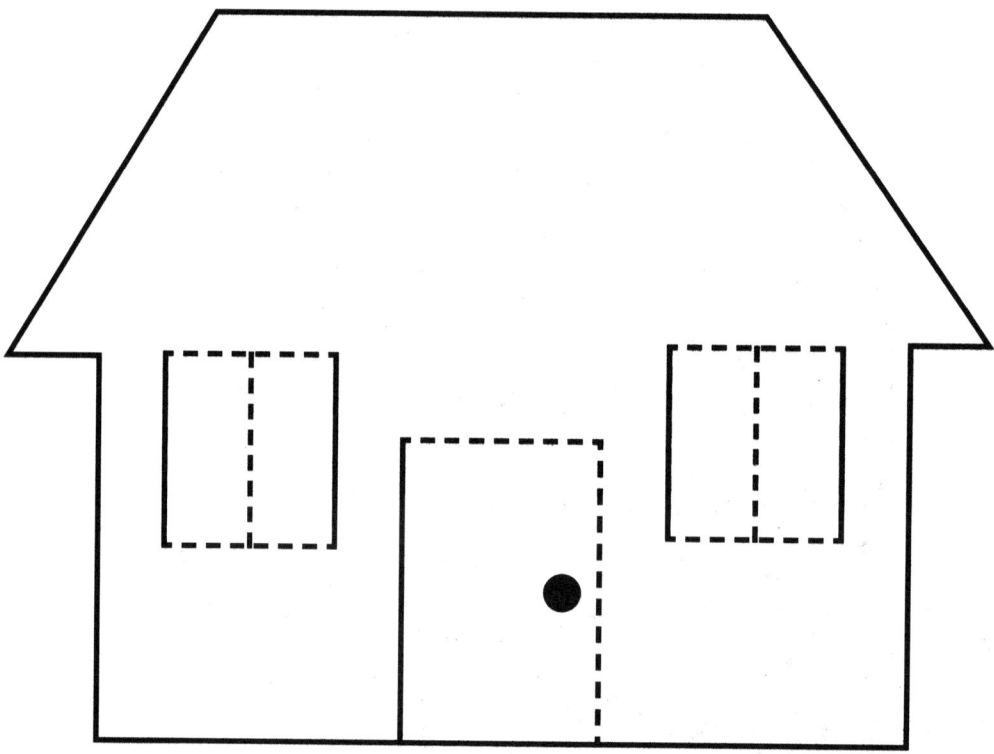

Worksheet 12

A flight of butterflies. This is an example of using paper folded concertina fashion to produce a string of figures. Care must be taken to leave the figures connected to each other. In this case this is achieved by the butterflies having flat sides to their upper wings. In the illustration below, cut along dotted lines, do not cut on the solid lines which indicate the folds of the paper.

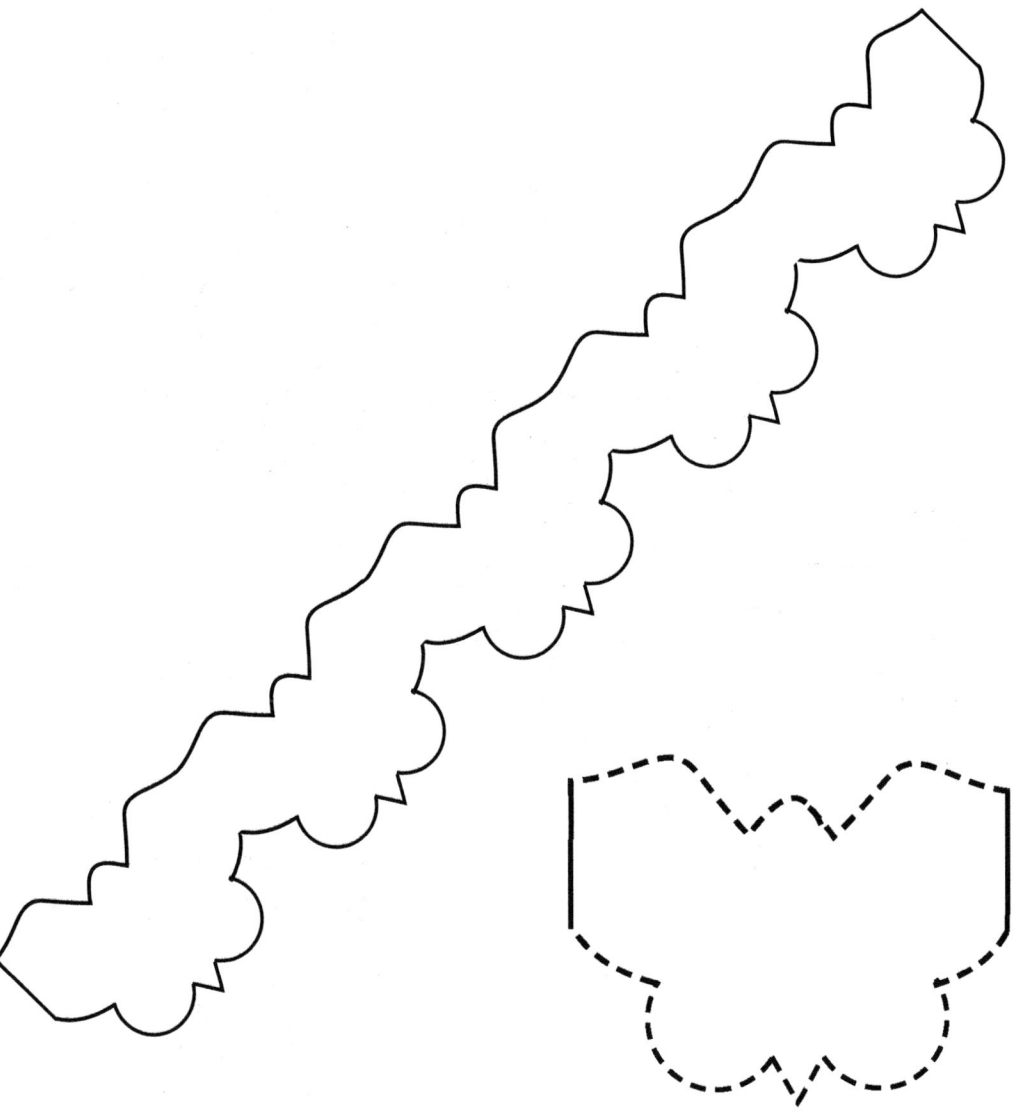

Worksheet 13

People holding hands. The figures may be further simplified or made more complex according to the maker's scissors skills. The ends of the arms must be aligned with folds of the paper and, of course, must not be cut.

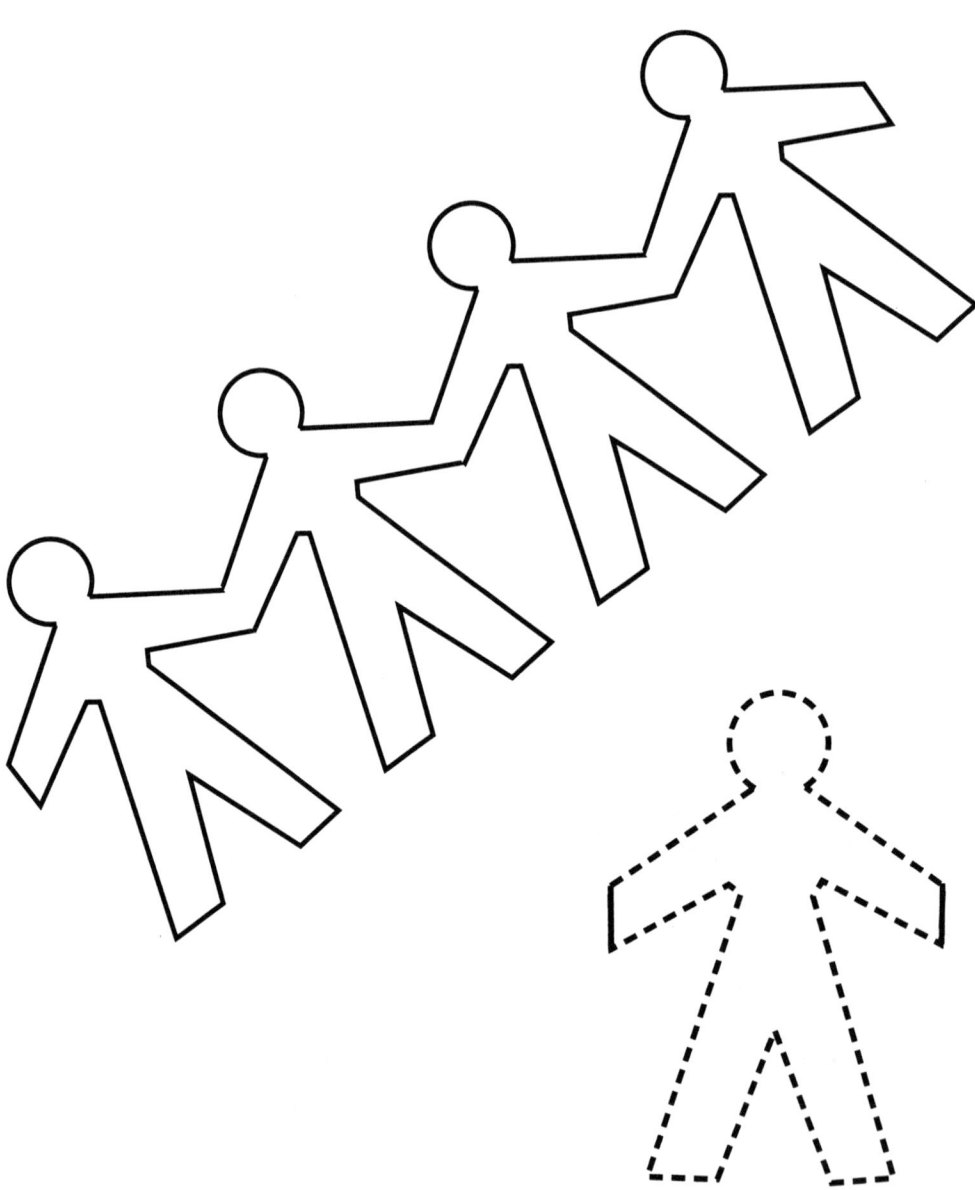

Worksheet 14

A simple flower shape cut from a circle of paper which was folded into quarters while it was being cut out. Such flowers made in various sizes using different colours and types of paper would make an attractive collage.

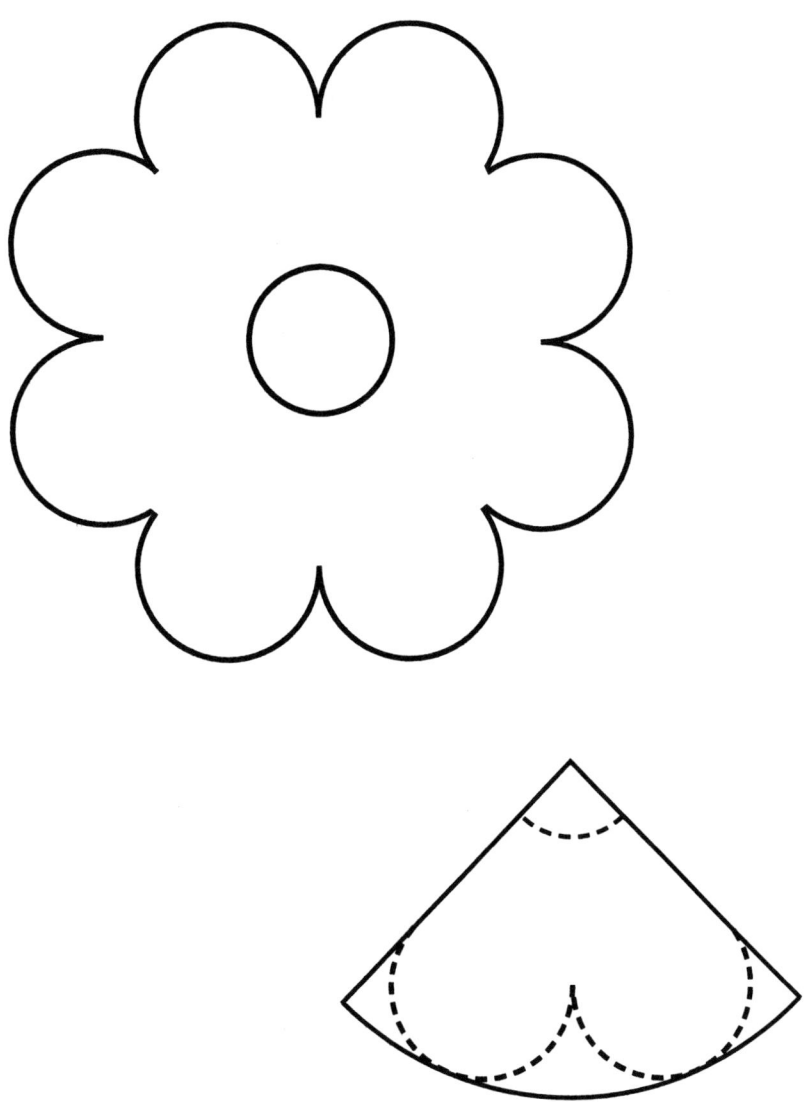

Worksheet 15

Examples of snowflake patterns cut from circles of paper. The circle for the pattern at the top of the page was folded into quarters and the one at the bottom of the page was folded into eighths before cutting. Those who are more skilled could make more complex and intricate patterns. Larger circles could be made into pretty doylies.

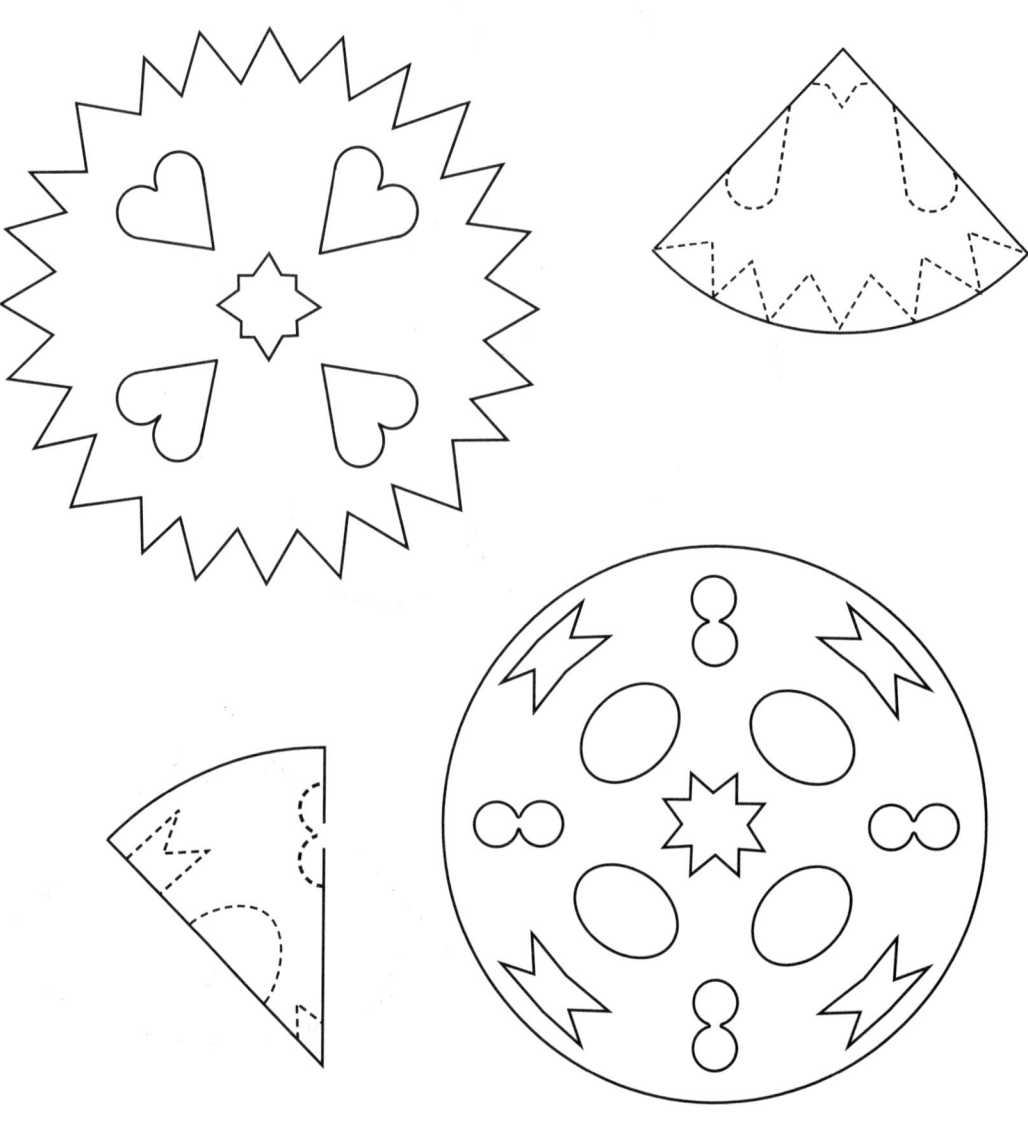

Worksheet 16

A greetings card made by layering simple card shapes one on top of the other. The 'sea' is three pieces of card, the edges cut with fancy craft scissors to simulate 'waves'. Each wave is accentuated with a little glitter glue. The boat is basically three triangles of card sitting in the 'waves'. The sun is a circle of gold refractive card and the greeting is from a sheet of peel-off greetings. All the card is attached with Sellotape self-adhesive Sticky Fixers which give a slightly three-dimensional effect.

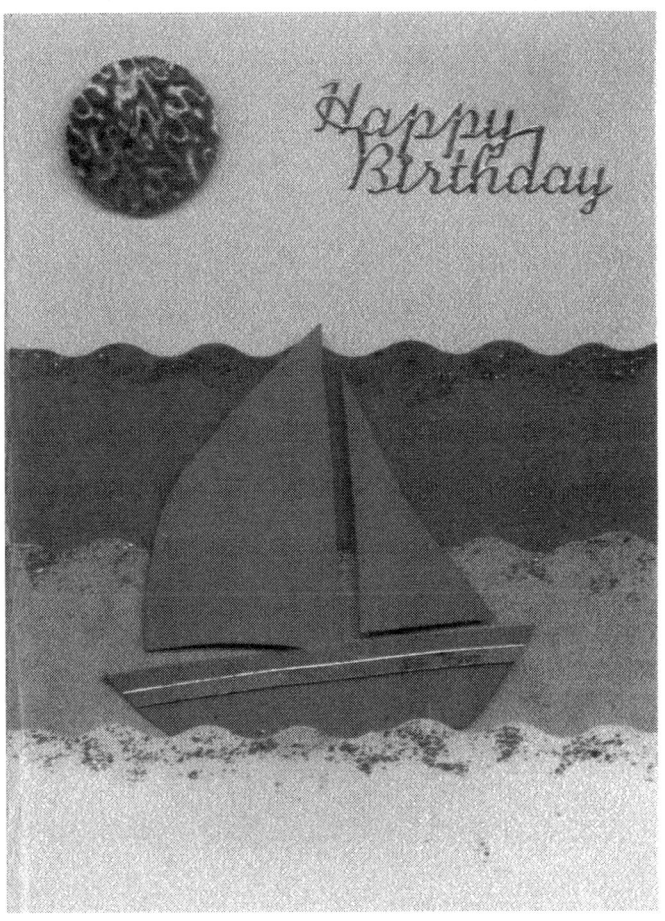

Worksheet 17

A quickly made greetings card using card and peel-off motifs. The card is of brown card on to which a square of corrugated metallic card is fixed. A smaller square of card is superimposed on the gold. The card is finished with peel-off motifs.

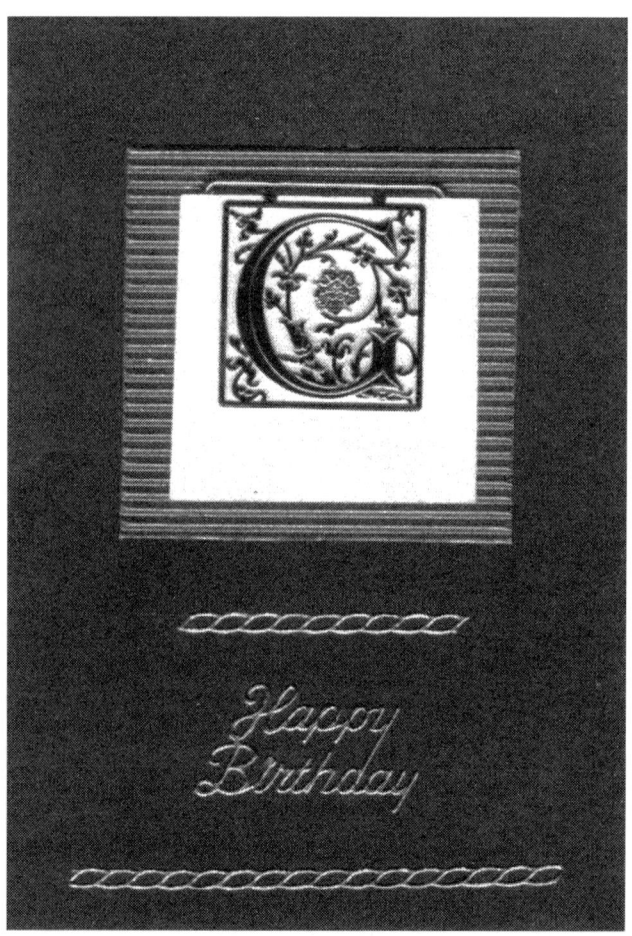

Worksheet 18

A greetings card using a variety of media. The card is made from burgundy card on which is superimposed a smaller piece of pink paper which has been cut with fancy craft scissors to produce a deckle edge. A 'jewel' is mounted on a strip of gold refractive card. A glitter pipe cleaner is fashioned into a heart shape with tails.

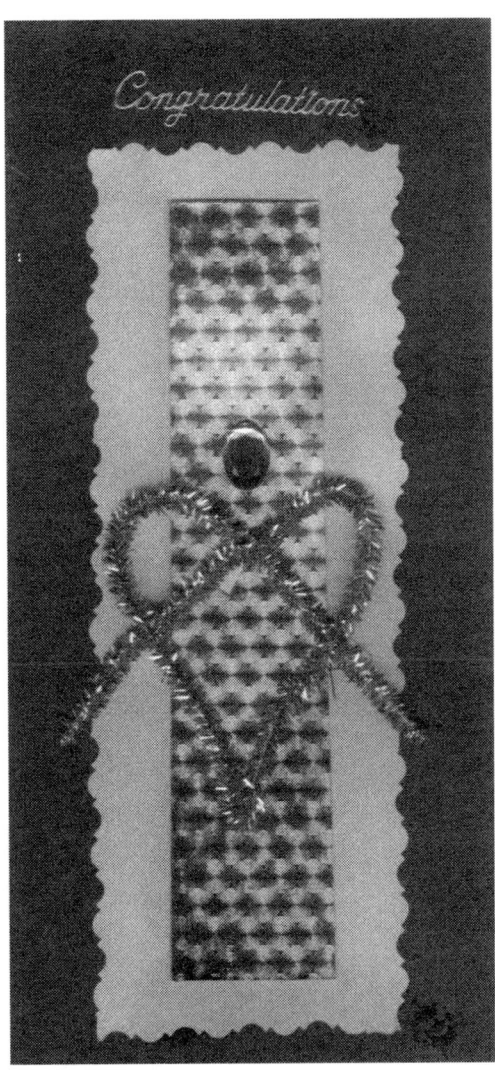

Index